Praise for *We Deserve More*

"Changing reproductive healthcare isn't just about policy—it's about culture, trust, and who gets heard. *We Deserve More* is a powerful example of how we can reach people in new ways, validate their experiences, and build confidence to demand better care. Nikki makes clear that patients' voices matter—and that expanding who tells these stories is how real change happens."

—Mini Timmaraju, President & CEO,
Reproductive Freedom for All

"*We Deserve More* truly captures how medical care can retraumatize us when compassion and consent are missing. Survivors already carry a lasting trauma; we deserve better care."

—Hadley Duvall, survivor and activist

"There's no question that our healthcare system is failing women when it comes to reproductive care, and this book opens your eyes to why you deserve so much better. Nikki weaves together her personal journey with hard truths about the system, drawing on her years of experience as a PA-C in women's health. What makes this book special is how she balances the big picture (calling out the systemic problems that hold us back) with practical advice you can use the next time you see your gynecologist. Her real-world experiences give weight to every recommendation, making this both an eye-opening critique and an empowering resource."

—Bayo Curry-Winchell, MD, MS, board-certified family
medicine physician and health advocate

"From over a decade of clinical experience as an OB/Gyn Physician Assistant, Nikki Sapiro Vinckier paints us a picture we cannot look away from— describing just how broken our reproductive health system is and the daily harms that system enacts on both patients and providers. Importantly, she compels us to go beyond anger and step into action, with concrete strategies to reshape and retake our reproductive health care into our own hands."

—Latona Giwa, Executive Director, Repro TLC

The We Deserve More Workbook

The We Deserve More Workbook

A Companion for Navigating Your Reproductive Healthcare

Nikki Sapiro Vinckier, PA-C

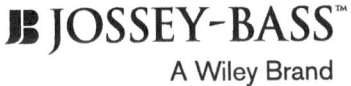
JOSSEY-BASS™
A Wiley Brand

Library of Congress Cataloging-in-Publication Data is available:

ISBN: 9781394416806 (Paperback)
ISBN: 9781394416813 (ePub)
ISBN: 9781394416820 (ePDF)

Cover Design: Wiley
Cover Image: © aminul788/stock.adobe.com
Author Photo: Purple Tree Photography

For every person who's ever left an appointment feeling small,
unheard, or like they were the problem.

You weren't.

You just deserved better care than the system was built to give you.

This is for everyone who's had to explain their pain twice,
for everyone who's been told to "just wait and see,"
for everyone who knew something was wrong and kept pushing anyway.

It's for the ones who still show up,
who still believe care can be better,
and who are learning to trust their voice again.

You deserve more than the bare minimum.

And this workbook will help you get it.

Contents

Introduction

Before You Begin

If you've ever walked out of a doctor's office feeling unheard, rushed, or unsure of what just happened, you're not alone. Maybe you spent the car ride over rehearsing your questions, only to lose them the moment you sat on the crinkly paper. Maybe you tried to describe your symptoms and got a shrug or a vague "let's just wait and see." Maybe you left with a prescription you weren't sure you wanted, or no plan at all.

Those moments don't just sting in the moment, they linger. They follow you home, into your group chats, into the quiet spaces where you wonder if you should even bother going back. They can shake your trust in the whole system, leaving you second-guessing not just your providers but also yourself. Did I explain it wrong? Did I not push hard enough? Am I the problem?

You're not the problem. The system is. And navigating it can feel complicated—sometimes routine, sometimes vulnerable, sometimes downright intimidating. You sit in the waiting room, clutching a clipboard full of forms, hoping the next 20 minutes will give you answers, or at least a plan. And too often, you leave with more questions than you came in with.

That's where this workbook comes in.

This isn't just another book to sit on your shelf. It's not a textbook or a journal you'll feel guilty for not finishing cover-to-cover. It's a living, breathing tool. A place to write, reflect, underline, and return to, before and after the appointments that shape your reproductive healthcare.

It was created to stand alongside my book, *We Deserve More: Why Reproductive Healthcare Is Broken—and What You Can Do About It.* The main book is where I break down the why: why the system looks the way it does, why it fails so many of us, and why it often feels like a battle just to get decent care. This workbook is where we shift to the how and what. How to prepare for a visit. How to advocate in the moment. How to recover when things don't go as planned. And how to walk back into care with a little more strength, confidence, and clarity than before. What symptoms you should track and what questions you should ask.

You can use this workbook in tandem with *We Deserve More,* flipping back and forth as you go. You can read that one first, let it sink in, and then come here when you're ready for the practical tools. Or you can pick this up on its own, without ever touching the other book, and still find a map for navigating your reproductive healthcare. There's no wrong way to use it.

Think of this as your personal manual. Your playbook. Your trusted companion in a system that doesn't always feel like it's on your side. You might keep it private. Scribbling in the margins, writing out scripts, tucking notes into the pages. Or you might decide to use it as something communal. Share it with a friend, a sister, a daughter, a partner. Pass it around your group chat like a repro workbook version of *The Sisterhood of the Traveling Pants.* Every time it lands in someone's hands, it brings a little more solidarity, a little more power. Because when one of us speaks up in a clinic or a hospital, it ripples out. And it makes space for others to do the same.

Our healthcare system is deeply flawed, but it's also the one we have to right now. This workbook won't replace your clinicians, and it certainly won't hand you every fact about every possible diagnosis. What it will do is give you a framework to step into your visits prepared, clear, and confident. It's here to help you make the most of the time you have with your clinicians. To help you ask sharper questions, to set boundaries, and to walk away with the information and support you need. You deserve care that works for you, even inside a system that doesn't always feel like it was built for you. This workbook is about making that possible. One visit at a time.

Two Parts, One Goal

The workbook is divided into two parts.

> **Part One** is Core Skills. These are the strategies that apply no matter who you are or what kind of visit you're walking into. They're the foundation: preparing for your annual exam, planning for a problem visit, asking better questions, bringing a support person, knowing how to push back, and knowing when it's time to walk away. These tools are your road map. They're here to help you turn a vague sense of "I hope this goes well" into a clear plan of action.
>
> **Part Two** is Real-Life Scenarios and Support. This is where we get into the specifics. The real-life situations that so many people face, but rarely have a manual for. What do you do if your teen is going to their first OB-GYN visit? How do you handle bias if your weight is the focus of the appointment instead of your actual concerns? What if you're navigating care as a Black woman, or as a trans or non-binary person, or with a history of trauma? What about irregular cycles, painful periods, infertility, miscarriage, abortion, or trying to build a family in ways medicine doesn't always explain? These scenarios aren't hypotheticals—they're the lived experiences that patients bring into exam rooms every day. And here, they come with scripts, checklists, reflection spaces, and prompts to help you find your footing.

The goal is not to overwhelm you with everything at once. The goal is to give you options, so that when you need them, the tools are already in your hands.

How to Use This Workbook

There's no right way to move through these pages. Some people will start at the beginning and go straight through. Others will flip directly to the scenario that matches what they're going through right now. That's the beauty of this format. Each section stands alone. You can skip, circle back, or revisit the same section multiple times as your life and needs change.

You can write in it. Highlight things that resonate. Copy a script onto a sticky note for your bag. Use the journaling prompts to sort through your thoughts before a visit. Tear out a page to bring to an appointment. Or just read and absorb, knowing that when you're in the exam room, the words might come back to you.

If you're someone who likes structure, you'll find checklists and templates to organize your medical story, track symptoms, or map out your next steps. If you're someone who processes through writing, there's space to journal and reflect. If you're someone who needs words in the moment, you'll find scripts you can borrow, adapt, or read verbatim. This book is here to meet you where you are.

Why It Matters

Reproductive healthcare in the United States is not designed to center patients. Appointments are short. Systems are rushed. Bias and dismissal are common. Too many people walk out of visits unheard, untreated, or worse—harmed.

But here's the other truth: when patients prepare, when we know our own needs, when we bring our questions and speak up, the balance of power shifts. Even if just a little. The system may be broken, but that doesn't mean you're powerless inside of it.

That's why this workbook exists. To give you concrete tools to bring your power into the exam room. To help you elevate your communication, your self-advocacy, and your sense of agency. To remind you that you're not asking for too much. You're asking for the basics: to be heard, respected, and cared for.

Beyond Gynecology: Where These Skills Go from Here

This workbook could go on forever. Because the truth is, what's broken in gynecology is just a reflection of what's broken across medicine. The short visits, the lack of listening, the gaps in communication, the way so many people walk out of care feeling unseen, those patterns show up everywhere.

But gynecology sits in a particularly charged space: the crosshairs of womanhood, patriarchy, and medicine. It's where centuries of bias about women's bodies, pain, and emotions still shape how care is delivered. It's where "normal" was defined by men who never lived inside these bodies. And it's where the lingering weight of those old systems still shows up in modern exam rooms, subtle but everywhere.

The skills you'll practice here don't stop at your annual exam or a visit with your OB-GYN. They apply anytime you interact with the medical system: at urgent care, in the emergency room, with a specialist or even at your child's pediatric appointment. Learning how to prepare, ask questions, and advocate for yourself doesn't just make gynecological care easier, it changes how you move through every kind of care.

But for this book, we'll stay right here. Focused on gynecology. Because this is where so many of us first learned how it feels to be dismissed, and where learning to take up space again can change everything. If you can build these skills in this room, you can take them anywhere.

You're Not Alone

Finally, I want to say this: however you choose to use this workbook, you're not alone in it. These pages are built on the experiences of countless patients who have walked through the same doors, asked the same questions, and faced the same dismissals. They've fought for better care. For themselves, for their families, and for others. You're part of that lineage now.

So take what you need from these pages. Use them as your prep kit before a vulnerable visit. Pass them along to a friend who's heading into something hard. Write in them late at night when you're trying to make sense of what happened at an appointment. Highlight the scripts that make your shoulders drop with relief. Carry the words with you into rooms that haven't always felt safe.

That's the heartbeat of this workbook. It won't fix the system overnight. I can't promise that you'll never have another frustrating visit. But this workbook exists to remind you that you have tools. You have power. And you deserve to walk into every exam room with tools and power. Because even when the system makes you feel small, your voice matters. Even when the appointment is rushed, your story is worth telling. And if the care falls short, may you always remember that you deserve more.

Part One

CORE SKILLS

Because every visit deserves both preparation and follow-through

This section is about building your foundation. It's about learning the skills that make visits smoother, clearer, and more empowering. Before we get into specific real-life scenarios, these pages focus on the abilities you can practice and strengthen over time: preparing before a visit, asking sharper questions, advocating in the moment, and following up after you leave.

Think of these skills as your road map. What to carry in with you and what to take away when you walk out. Preparation matters. Gathering your questions, tracking your symptoms, setting boundaries, and knowing what you want from the visit changes everything once you're in the room.

But the truth is, a visit doesn't end when you leave the room. Results need to come back. Referrals need to happen. Prescriptions need to get filled. Sometimes even your own feelings about how it went need space to land. The skills you build before and after are what help move your care forward while keeping your needs at the center.

Each skill stands on its own, so you can jump to what you need most. Maybe it's organizing your story and symptoms before you go. Maybe it's finding the words to push back in real time. Maybe it's regrouping afterward if things didn't go the way you hoped.

These aren't extras. They're essentials. They're the quiet, often-untaught abilities that make your visits more productive and your care more collaborative. The system doesn't make it easy, and learning these skills can change how you move through it.

These pages are your guideposts. Your anchor. The starting point for every kind of care. They're applicable far beyond just your reproductive care. Because no matter what brings you into the exam room—or what lingers after—you deserve to be prepared, supported, and heard.

Skill 1

Your Medical Snapshot

In today's healthcare system, you can't count on every provider, or every appointment, to hold the whole picture of who you are and what you've been through. Records get lost, systems don't talk to each other, and rushed visits mean important details can slip through the cracks. That's why one of the most powerful things you can do as a patient is to keep your own version of your medical story.

This isn't about documenting a perfect medical record, that's your clinicians job. This is about giving yourself something much more practical: a snapshot you can carry into the room, use as a quick reference in the moment, and look back on later when you're planning follow-up or preparing for the next visit.

Think of it as your personal anchor. When nerves or "white coat brain" kick in, you don't have to rely on memory. When you're juggling multiple doctors, specialists, or follow-ups, you have one place to keep your history straight. When you want to make sure your top concerns don't get lost in the shuffle, you already have them written down.

Your medical story is also the foundation of your advocacy. In today's world, you have to be your own best advocate. And that advocacy starts with knowing the details of your health and healthcare history. By writing them down on your terms, you control the narrative. You decide what matters most. You make it easier for yourself to speak up, and harder for anyone else to overlook what's important to you.

This tool helps you start building that foundation. Use it before every visit, keep it in your bag or on your phone, and tuck it into your larger care folder if you're creating one. Over time, it becomes not just a reference sheet, but a running record of your health story. Focusing on the version that puts you and your experience at the center.

What to Include

Your medical story doesn't need to be exhaustive to be useful. The goal isn't to capture every detail of your life, it's to have the essentials at your fingertips so you can walk into any appointment feeling clear and prepared. Think of this as your quick reference sheet but also the starting point for your care folder.

My Care Snapshot

This is a quick-reference sheet to bring into visits. Fill in what matters most, no need to capture everything.

The Basics

- Name/pronouns/date of birth: _____
- Emergency contact (optional): _____
- Preferred pharmacy (name, address, phone): _____

Current Medications and Supplements

(List prescriptions, over-the-counter meds, vitamins, herbs, doses and frequency, and then if it differs, how you actually take them.)

_____

_____

_____

Allergies

(Medications, foods, or environmental allergens and your reaction.)

_____

_____

_____

Medical and Surgical History

(Past diagnoses or surgeries. Add the year if you recall.)

_____

_____

_____

OB-GYN History (If Relevant)

☐ Pregnancies/births _____

☐ Miscarriages/abortions _____

☐ Menstrual/menopause status _____

☐ Conditions (fibroids, polycystic ovary syndrome [PCOS], endometriosis) _____

Family History

(Major conditions that run in your family—cancers, diabetes, blood clots, heart disease.)

_____

_____

_____

My Priorities for This Visit

(Top one to two things that I want addressed today, plus boundaries or requests.)

_____

_____

_____

Provider Directory

- Primary care: _____
- OB-GYN: _____
- Specialists: _____
- Pharmacy: _____

Key Results

(Any Notable Recent Labs / Tests)

_____

_____

_____

Symptom Snapshot

(Main symptoms, triggers, what helps. See Skill 5 for tracking your symptoms.)

_____

_____

_____

Preferences and Boundaries

- ☐ I want clear explanations before procedures.
- ☐ I want pain management offered for in-office procedures.
- ☐ I prefer a support person present for pelvic exams.
- ☐ Other: _____

Emergency and Safety Notes

(Critical information for urgent care—for example, allergies, blood thinners, past ectopic.)

_____

_____

Insurance and Coverage Snapshot

- Plan/identification number: _____
- Copay/deductible notes: _____
- Any other coverage/benefits to note: _____

Future Care Goals

- Short term (next three to six months): _____
- Long term (family planning, menopause care, mental health, etc.): _____

  _____

Reflection Prompts

- What do I usually forget to bring up in visits?

- What matters most to me right now—even if it feels small?

- If I only had three minutes with my provider, what would I make sure gets said?

Key Takeaway

This is your story, on your terms. Filling it out once gives you a baseline. Updating it over time turns it into a care folder you can carry with you. One that keeps you prepared, organized, and in control no matter where your healthcare journey takes you.

Skill 2

Making the Right Appointment: Setting Yourself Up for Success

One of the biggest hidden frustrations in healthcare happens before you even see your provider. You call to schedule, but the scheduler asks, "Is this for your annual?" You say yes, because it seems right. Maybe you haven't been in a year. But after your visit you walk out frustrated because the reason why you called in the first place, your problem, wasn't even addressed. Or you come in ready for a procedure, only to find it wasn't scheduled correctly and you have to come back another day.

Here's an important truth that many people don't know: not all appointments are the same. And knowing which kind you need will save you time, money, and a lot of frustration.

The Main Appointment Types

Knowing what kind of visit you're booking makes all the difference. Each appointment type has its own purpose, time allotment, and billing rules. If you walk in expecting one thing but the office has you scheduled for another, you'll often leave frustrated—or worse, told to come back.

- **Preventive visits** (annual exams) are designed for check-ups and screenings when you're otherwise healthy.
- **Problem-focused visits** are for one main issue you need answers on.
- **Procedure visits** are exactly what they sound like—specific in-office procedures.
- **Counseling or extended visits** (if your clinic offers them) give you more time to dive into complex concerns.

Why this matters: If you book an annual but want to talk about infertility, you'll leave disappointed. If you expect an intrauterine device (IUD) at a problem visit, you may be told, "We can't do that today." If you don't request extended time, your provider may only have 10 minutes for something that really needs 30.

How to Help Yourself When You Call

Schedulers often default to "annual exam" unless you specify otherwise. When you call, be clear about what you want from the visit, ask what appointment types are available, and confirm before hanging up. Use simple language like the following:

- "I'd like to schedule my annual preventive exam."
- "I need a problem-focused visit for heavy bleeding that's affecting my daily life."
- "I'd like to schedule an IUD placement. Can you confirm it's booked as a procedure so it's actually placed that day?"
- "I'd like an appointment for fertility planning, and I think I'll need extra time. Is there an option for extended counseling?"

Think of it like ordering from a menu: you'll get the right thing only if you call it by name.

Quick Reference Chart

Type of Visit	Best For	Not For	What to Say When You Call	Billing/Pro Tips
Preventive (annual)	Screenings, Pap smear, vaccines, family/medical history updates, quick medication refills	Ongoing problems (pain, infertility, heavy bleeding, chronic concerns)	"I'd like to schedule my annual preventive exam."	Usually covered in full by insurance (no copay)

Problem-focused	One main issue: pain, bleeding, discharge, fertility, mood changes, sexually transmitted infection testing	Multiple unrelated problems or preventive screenings	"I'd like a problem-focused visit for ___."	Copay/deductible may apply
Procedure	IUD insertion, biopsy, colposcopy, ultrasound	General discussion or counseling	"I need a procedure visit for ___."	**Pro tip.** Confirm it's scheduled correctly or you may be told to rebook. May need pre-authorization; copay/coinsurance possible
Counseling/extended	Fertility planning, menopause management, hormone therapy, trauma-focused care	Quick check-ins or routine refills	"I'd like an extended counseling visit for ___."	Often billed as problem-focused but coded for longer time

Pro tip. Procedures require the right room, staff, and setup. Always double-check that it's scheduled for your procedure, not just a regular problem visit.

Insurance reminder. Preventive visits are usually covered with no copay, but if you raise a new problem at that visit, it may be billed separately and you could see a charge.

Reflection Prompts

- Have I ever booked the wrong type of appointment without realizing it?

- What kind of visit do I actually need right now?

- How confident do I feel asking for what I need when I call?

Worksheet: My Appointment Plan

1. What's bringing me in?

(Check one that feels most true, or add your own.)

- ☐ I'm due for my annual check-up (screenings, Pap, vaccines).
- ☐ I have one main concern I want addressed (pain, bleeding, fertility, mood, discharge).
- ☐ I need a specific procedure (IUD placement, biopsy, colposcopy, ultrasound).
- ☐ I want more in-depth counseling (fertility planning, menopause, hormone therapy, trauma-focused care).
- ☐ Other: _____

2. If I could only accomplish one thing at this visit, it would be ...

(Write your top priority in one sentence. Example: "I want to get answers about my heavy bleeding" or "I want to have my IUD placed.")

_____

_____

3. What outcome am I hoping for?

(Check all that apply)

- ☐ A diagnosis or explanation
- ☐ A prescription or medication change
- ☐ A procedure or device placed
- ☐ A referral to a specialist
- ☐ Counseling, education, or reassurance
- ☐ Other: _____

4. How will I say it when I call?

Write your one-sentence request here:

"I'd like to schedule ... _____."

5. What do I need to double-check before hanging up?

- ☐ The appointment type matches what I need (preventive, problem-focused, procedure, extended).
- ☐ The billing category is what I expect (preventive versus problem-focused).
- ☐ If it's a procedure, that it's actually scheduled to happen that day.

Skill 3

Preparing for Your Annual Exam

An annual exam is meant to be about prevention. Think of it like routine maintenance for your body. You're checking in before something feels wrong, making sure screenings are up-to-date, and giving yourself a chance to ask general questions about your health. In theory, it should feel thorough and reassuring. In reality, it often feels rushed, awkward, or impersonal.

One of the biggest sources of frustration around annual exams comes from mismatched expectations. Many people show up hoping to address specific symptoms or ongoing concerns, only to leave feeling unheard when those issues aren't fully addressed. That experience can feel dismissive, even when no one intended it to be.

This section will help you make the most of your annual exam by understanding what it's for, how to prepare, and what you can reasonably expect. In the next skill, we'll talk about how to book and plan visits when you do have something specific you need addressed.

What Your Annual Exam Is (and Isn't)

An annual exam is best for the following issues:
- Updating your medical history
- Reviewing medications and allergies

- Checking on preventive screenings (Pap smears, mammograms, blood work, vaccines)
- Discussing general wellness (sleep, cycle, sexual health, mood)
- Raising one to two smaller concerns or questions

It is not the best time for the following issues:
- In-depth conversations about ongoing problems (like chronic pain, infertility, or heavy bleeding)
- Complex issues that need testing or procedures
- Extended counseling (like detailed fertility planning, trauma processing, or hormone therapy discussions)

Why? Because annual visits are scheduled and billed as preventive care. They're set up to be a broad overview, not a deep dive. If you try to cover too much, you'll likely feel rushed—or worse, important issues get brushed off and remain unaddressed.

If you have a deeper or more urgent concern, the best thing you can do for yourself is to book a problem-focused visit. That doesn't mean you can't mention a concern during your annual, it just means you'll get better, more focused care if you schedule the right kind of appointment for your needs.

Healthcare in America is a game, and unfortunately you need to know how to play by the rules to get what you need from it.

A Note About OB-GYNs and Primary Care

One important reality to consider: many people use their OB-GYN as their primary care provider (PCP). It makes sense in some ways, you might see your OB-GYN more often than any other clinician, and the relationship can feel comfortable and familiar. But here's the truth: OB-GYNs shouldn't be responsible for everything, and you may be short-changing yourself if you lean on them to manage your whole health picture.

OB-GYNs are experts in reproductive health. Their training is specialized in pregnancy, gynecologic health, contraception, menopause, and preventive care like Pap smears and breast exams. Yes, they can order basic labs like cholesterol panels, blood sugar, and thyroid tests. Yes, they can check your blood pressure and renew certain prescriptions. But managing long-term conditions like hypertension, high cholesterol, diabetes, asthma, or thyroid disease isn't really within their wheelhouse.

Why does this matter? Because chronic conditions need ongoing monitoring, medication adjustments, and coordination with other specialists. That's the job of a

PCP, a family medicine doctor, internal medicine doctor, nurse practitioner, or physician assistant trained to look at the whole person, not just reproductive health.

If you rely on your OB-GYN alone, things can slip through the cracks. For example:

- Your OB-GYN may order a cholesterol panel but not adjust your medications or track your numbers every few months.
- They may note that your blood pressure is high but not initiate or titrate treatment.
- They may refill your asthma inhaler but not check your lung function or long-term control.

This is not about blaming providers. It is about understanding the system well enough to use it safely. Going to the wrong person for the wrong concern does not just slow things down. It increases the risk of fragmented care and leaves patients feeling unheard when what they really needed was a different type of visit or provider.

Reflecting on Where Your Needs Belong

When you prepare for your annual, take a minute to reflect on these questions:

- Are my concerns mostly about reproductive health (periods, birth control, pregnancy, menopause, sexual health)? OB-GYN is the right place.

- Do I have chronic conditions that need monitoring (high blood pressure, diabetes, cholesterol, thyroid disease)? These are best managed by a PCP.

- Am I due for general preventive care (like colonoscopy, skin checks, or vaccinations outside of reproductive health)? Your PCP is the one who keeps track of these and refers you to the right specialists—for example, gastrointestinal for colonoscopy, dermatology for skin checks, or pharmacy/clinic for vaccines if they don't have them available.

Having both an OB-GYN and a PCP is ideal. The OB-GYN can focus on your reproductive and gynecologic care while your PCP manages your broader health needs and makes sure the rest of your preventive care doesn't fall through the cracks. The two should complement, not replace, each other.

If you don't have a PCP, your OB-GYN may be able to give you a referral. It's worth asking: "Do you think I should establish care with a primary care provider for my general health needs?"

The Bottom Line

Your annual exam is valuable, but it has limits. If you prepare ahead and know what fits into that visit, you'll leave with more of your priorities covered. And if some concerns belong with a primary care provider instead, that's not a failure, it's part of building a full team for your health. When each provider is doing the work they're trained for, you get better, safer, and more thorough care.

How to Prepare for Your Annual

1. **Update your medical snapshot** (see Skill 1).
2. **Write down your top priorities**, but know you'll likely only have time for one or two.
3. **Bring your cycle details** (first day of your last period, changes in bleeding or pain).
4. **Review your screenings.** Know when your last Pap, mammogram, colonoscopy, or labs were done so you can ask if you're due. If they were done at a different office have the results available. Screenshots work fine.
5. **Set your expectations.** Are my needs "annual exam" appropriate or do they deserve their own problem visit?

Questions to Ask at Your Annual Exam

- "Am I up-to-date on all my screenings for my age and history?"
- "Are there preventive steps I should be thinking about right now (vaccines, labs, lifestyle)?"
- "Does my family history change which screenings I should get and/or frequency?"
- "Can we review my medications to make sure they're still the best fit?"
- "Are there concerns I should take to a PCP instead of my OB-GYN?"

Prioritizing Your Concerns

Use your annual exam to get clarity on *prevention and maintenance*, and to surface small concerns you don't want ignored. But if something is bigger, ongoing, or seriously affecting your quality of life, schedule a problem visit.

You deserve enough time for the things that matter most.

Reflection Prompts

- What's one thing I want to make sure gets covered at my next annual?

- Have I ever tried to squeeze a big problem into an annual exam? How did that go?

- What would it look like to give myself permission to book a problem visit when I need one?

- If my OB-GYN is the only doctor I see regularly, what might be falling through the cracks?

Quick Checklist Before You Go

☐ Updated medical snapshot is ready.
☐ My top concerns for this annual exam:

_____

_____

_____

☐ My cycle info:
  - Date of last period: _____
  - Or menopause status: _____
  - Regular cycle: Yes/no
  - Typical cycle duration (from first day of one cycle to first day of next cycle):

    _____

☐ Most recent screening dates and results if it wasn't normal:
  - Pap smear: _____
  - Mammogram: _____
  - Colonoscopy: _____
  - Blood work/labs: _____
  - Other: _____

☐ Any must-ask questions:

_____

_____

_____

_____

Skill 4

Planning for a Problem Visit

When something is bothering you, like pain, bleeding, or a change in your body, you deserve a visit that gives it the attention it needs. Unlike an annual exam, which is broad and preventive, a problem visit zeroes in on one main concern.

Too often, patients show up with a laundry list of issues and leave feeling like none of them got addressed. Or they bring up something complicated at the very end of a rushed annual and are told, "We'll need another appointment." Choosing the right type of visit (see Skill 2) is the first step. The second is coming prepared, clear, and confident.

What a problem visit is for:

- One specific issue (like pelvic pain, heavy bleeding, fertility concerns, urinary symptoms)
- New or worsening symptoms
- Ongoing problems that haven't been resolved
- Conversations that require more depth than an annual exam allows
- In-depth medication management or prescription changes

It's not for:

- Covering multiple unrelated issues
- Preventive screenings (Pap smears, mammogram, labs—that's annual exam territory)
- Long counseling sessions (unless you set that expectation when scheduling)

Reflection Prompts Before Your Visit

- What symptom or issue do I want this visit to focus on?

- How has this been affecting my daily life?

- What do I most want to walk away with: answers, a plan, testing, or a referral?

How to Frame Your Symptoms Clearly

When time is short, clarity matters. Providers often think in patterns—what started when, what makes it better or worse, and how it's affecting your life. You want to get good at sharing a focused snapshot.

Try using this framework:

Symptom. What's happening? (e.g., pelvic pain, irregular bleeding)
Timeline. When did it start? How often does it happen?
Triggers/patterns. Do you notice what makes it better or worse?
What you've tried. Any meds, lifestyle changes, or treatments you've already attempted.
Impact. How is it affecting your daily life? (work, sleep, sex, activities)

Example: "I've had pelvic pain for about six months. It's worse during my period and after sex. I've tried ibuprofen, but it doesn't help. It's making it hard to get through work."

The next tool will walk you through tracking all this in more detail.

Advocating If You're Brushed Off

Sometimes, providers minimize symptoms—especially pain, bleeding, or hormonal concerns. If you get brushed off, here are quick scripts you can lean on:

- **If told it's "normal."** "I hear you, but it doesn't feel normal for me. Can you explain why you're not concerned?"
- **If redirected too quickly.** "I'd like to make sure we spend time on this today. This is the reason I came in. Can you help me understand what tests or next steps we should take?"
- **If you're told to just wait it out.** "What signs would tell you this needs more urgent attention? I'd like a plan if either it doesn't improve or gets worse."
- **If you need a referral.** "Is this something that you routinely manage, or do I need a different clinician/specialist?"

Worksheet: My Problem Visit Snapshot

Main issue I want addressed: _____

My top three questions for this visit:

1. _____

2. _____

3. _____

What I need most today:
- ☐ Reassurance/clarity
- ☐ Testing/labs
- ☐ Treatment options
- ☐ Referral to specialist
- ☐ Next steps/timeline

Skill 5

Tracking Symptoms

Even with the best intentions, it's hard to remember details when you're sitting on the exam table. You might have been dealing with something for weeks, or even months, but when asked "When did this start?" or "How often does it happen?" it's easy to go blank.

That's why tracking your symptoms ahead of time can help. A simple log gives you a clear picture of what's happening so you don't have to rely on memory alone. You'll walk into your appointment prepared, focused, and confident that you have the details ready when you need them.

Why Symptom Tracking Helps

- **It shows patterns.** Documenting when and how symptoms occur gives clinicians critical diagnostic information. For example, pelvic pain and gastrointestinal pain can overlap and mimic each other. Tracking the timing, context, and triggers of your pain helps clarify whether it is more likely gynecologic, gastrointestinal, or a combination of both. This makes it easier for your clinician to direct you toward the right evaluation and treatment. Just as important, having this record reduces the chance of your concerns being dismissed. It establishes that you know your body, have observed it carefully, and are coming prepared with evidence that deserves attention.

- **It highlights severity.** Many people normalize pain or discomfort over time, convincing themselves it is "not that bad." Writing down how severe symptoms feel, using a 1 to 10 scale or descriptive terms, creates a record that better reflects the true intensity of what you're experiencing. This helps clinicians differentiate between mild, moderate, and severe conditions, and it supports more accurate decisions about treatment.
- **It proves impact.** Symptoms are often minimized until their real-life consequences are clear. By recording how often symptoms interfere with sleep, work, caregiving, exercise, or relationships, you demonstrate the toll they take on your daily functioning. This evidence shows that the issue is not just uncomfortable, but disruptive. And it needs to be taken seriously.
- **It keeps you focused.** In the moment, it can be difficult to recall details or explain them clearly. A written log prevents that. Instead of struggling to remember timelines or drifting into vague descriptions, you can present a concise, fact-based account of what has been happening. This ensures your limited appointment time is used effectively and that your key concerns are addressed.

When you show up with documented evidence, you demonstrate that you know and understand your body. It makes it harder for your concerns to be dismissed or gaslit, and it shifts the encounter into a more collaborative space. A space where your experience is respected, and your clinician can better work with you to find answers and solutions.

What to Track

You do not need to log every aspect of your daily routine, but you do need to track the details that give a clinician a complete picture of your symptoms. Accuracy and consistency matter. The following categories are the most important to record:

Date. Note the day symptoms occurred. This helps establish patterns over time.
Symptom. Name what's happening in your own words. Don't worry about sounding "medical." Just describe it the way you feel it.

- Examples: pelvic pain, cramping, irregular bleeding, bloating, hot flashes, headaches, fatigue, low mood, anxiety, unusual discharge, urinary urgency.
- If you have multiple symptoms, note whether they always appear together or come and go separately.

Severity. This shows how disruptive the symptom really is.

- Use a 1–10 scale (1 = barely noticeable, 10 = unbearable).
- Or, stick with words: mild, moderate, severe.
- If the symptom fluctuates, track both the "average" and the "worst it gets."
- Sometimes it helps to describe what each level means for you (e.g., *"A 7 means I had to leave work early"*).

Duration/timing. Clarity about timing helps providers see patterns.

- When did this first start?
- How long does each episode last—minutes, hours, days?
- How often does it happen—daily, weekly, only around your period, only with certain activities?
- Is it constant, or does it come and go?

Patterns/triggers. Even small observations here can be gold for your provider.

- Do you notice symptoms around your period, with stress, after certain foods, or during exercise?
- Does it get worse at a certain time of day?
- Does activity, rest, position changes, or certain medications make it better or worse?
- Do hormones, sex, or bladder/bowel changes seem to play a role?

Impact on life. This is where symptoms stop being abstract and show how they really affect you.

- Does it interrupt sleep?
- Keep you from work, school, or caregiving?
- Make exercise, sex, or daily activities harder?
- Affect your mood or relationships?
- Cause you to avoid things you normally enjoy?

What you've tried (and what helps, if anything). This is about two things: showing what you've already attempted so your provider doesn't just suggest the same first steps again, and identifying whether anything makes a difference, even temporarily. By capturing both the *attempt* and the *result*, you give your provider a much clearer picture of what's been tried, what can be ruled out, and where to focus next.

- **Medications.** Prescription or over-the-counter. Note how you actually take them (e.g., "Ibuprofen 400 mg once a day" or "birth control pill, but I sometimes miss doses").
- **Lifestyle changes.** Adjustments to diet, exercise, hydration, caffeine, alcohol, or sleep.
- **Comfort measures.** Heat pads, ice packs, baths, rest, massage, topical creams, relaxation techniques.
- **Complementary approaches.** Supplements, acupuncture, chiropractic care, pelvic floor physical therapy, counseling, or other nontraditional strategies.
- **Effectiveness.** Did it help? Not at all? A little bit? Made it worse? For example: "Ibuprofen dulls it for a couple of hours, but doesn't make it go away."
- **Side effects.** Did the treatment itself cause problems—like nausea, drowsiness, or mood changes?

Sample Symptom Log

Date	Symptom	Severity (1–10)	Duration/ Timing	Patterns/ Triggers	Impact on Life	What I Tried
May 3	Pelvic pain	7	2 hours, mid-morning	Started 2 days before period; worse after lunch	Couldn't finish work project; skipped workout	Ibuprofen 400 mg, heat pad (only slight relief)
May 4	Pelvic pain	8	4 hours, all afternoon	On period day 1; standing made it worse	Left work early; hard to sleep later	Ibuprofen 600 mg, hot shower (helped briefly)
May 6	Pelvic pain	6	1 hour, evening	Period tapering; pain less severe	Managed normal tasks but felt drained	Rested, no meds

(Notice how this gives a clear picture: timing, severity, impact, what helped or didn't. That's exactly what your provider needs to see patterns.)

Now make your own:

Date	Symptom	Severity (1–10)	Duration/ Timing	Patterns/ Triggers	Impact on Life	What I Tried

Reflection Prompts

- What patterns do I notice now that I can see my symptoms mapped out over time?

- How do these symptoms interfere with the parts of life that matter most to me (work, family, relationships, sleep, daily functioning)?

- What changes or triggers stand out when I compare good days and bad days?

- What treatments, medications, or strategies seemed to help, even a little, and what made things worse?

- How does having this written record change the way I feel about my symptoms and my ability to talk about them?

- If my provider only had three minutes, what are the top facts I would want them to understand from my log?

Worksheet: My Simple Symptom Snapshot (Quick Version)

If you didn't have time to keep a detailed symptom log, use this quick worksheet before your visit. It captures the essentials your clinician needs to understand what's happening.

Main symptom I want to discuss: _____

When it happens/how often: _____

How severe it feels at its worst (*circle*): 1　2　3　4　5　6　7　8　9　10

How severe it feels at baseline (*circle*): 1　2　3　4　5　6　7　8　9　10

How it affects my daily life (*check all that apply and write down any pertinent details*):

- ☐ Missed work/school
- ☐ Interrupted sleep
- ☐ Limited activities/exercise
- ☐ Affected relationships/sex life
- ☐ Emotional strain (stress, frustration, sadness)
- ☐ Other: _____

What I've tried so far (and whether it helped): _____

What I want to ask my provider about this: _____

_____

Tips for Success

- Don't overthink it. Even jotting a few notes in your phone is enough.
- Consistency beats detail. A few weeks of light tracking is more valuable than trying to capture every single moment.
- Use your words. Write it the way you experience it. There's no need to sound "medical."
- Bring it with you. On paper, in your phone, or even as a photo. Just make sure you can reference it during your visit.

Skill 6

The Art of Good Questions

Time with a provider is limited, often just a few minutes. In those moments, the way you ask a question can shape the entire visit. A closed question like "Is this normal?" usually gets you a one-word answer. An open question like "What could be causing this?" invites your provider to explain, think out loud, and share options you might not otherwise hear.

Good questions aren't about sounding like a doctor or using medical terms. They're about creating clarity and opening doors for conversation, education, and collaboration. The right question can turn a vague reassurance into a concrete explanation, a rushed dismissal into a thoughtful plan, or a confusing test result into something you actually understand.

This is where power shifts. Instead of being a passive recipient of care, you become an active partner in the process. You're guiding the conversation toward what matters most: clear information, real options, and next steps that you can act on. And when you know how to ask well, you leave with more than just answers. You leave with a plan.

Why Questions Matter

- **They shift the dynamic.** Asking thoughtful questions moves you from a passive role into an active one. You are not simply receiving information, you are shaping the direction of the visit.
- **They bring clarity.** Medical shorthand can leave patients in the dark. Instead of hearing "Your labs are fine," a good follow-up question might get you "Your blood sugar is 92, which falls in the normal range. If it were over 100, we'd begin to discuss pre-diabetes." The difference between vague reassurance and precise information is the difference between confusion and understanding.
- **They prevent dismissal.** Too often, symptoms—especially pain, bleeding, or hormonal concerns—are minimized. Direct questions about cause, risk, or next steps make it harder for a provider to move on without addressing your concern. When you ask, "What could this mean if it doesn't improve?" or "What red flags should I watch for?" you are establishing that your symptoms deserve attention, not dismissal.
- **They create a plan.** A good question doesn't just get you an answer, it sets the stage for what comes next. Whether it's deciding on a test, weighing treatment options, or agreeing on follow-up, questions are the tool that turns a short visit into a road map for your care.

Types of Questions That Get Results

Open-Ended Questions
These invite explanations instead of a yes/no answer. They encourage your provider to share more detail and give you a fuller picture.
- "What could be causing this?"
- "What options do I have for treating this?"
- "How will we know if this is working?"

Clarifying Questions
These push vague statements into specific, useful information. They prevent you from leaving the visit with only half an answer.
- "When you say it's 'normal,' what do you mean?"
- "Can you walk me through what you're looking for in this exam?"

Next-Step Questions

These make sure the visit ends with a clear plan. They establish what to do if things don't improve and when to follow up.

- "What happens if this doesn't get better?"
- "When should I come back, and what would trigger a sooner follow-up?"

Options and Trade-Offs Questions

These help you weigh risks and benefits so you can make informed decisions.

- "If we don't treat this now, what are the risks?"
- "What's the difference between these two medications?"

Partnership Questions

These show you are engaged in your care and invite collaboration. They remind your provider that you want to work as a team.

- "What do you need from me to help figure this out?"
- "How can I track my symptoms so it's useful for you?"

Insider Tip: Ask for the Differential

A *differential diagnosis* is the list of possible explanations a clinician keeps in mind when evaluating your symptoms. It's the mental map they use to consider what might be going on, what's most likely, and what needs to be ruled out.

Why do this? Because it pushes the conversation deeper. It brings potential risks or conditions into the open, and makes your provider explain their reasoning, and ensures your concerns are taken seriously. It shifts the interaction from vague reassurance to a transparent, collaborative process—so you leave knowing what's on the table and how it will be addressed.

When you ask about the differential, you're really saying, "Don't stop at the first idea. Walk me through the other possibilities. Help me understand what you're considering, and why."

For example, instead of hearing only, "Your bleeding is normal," you might hear, "This could be related to a polyp, hormonal changes, or something structural like fibroids. Based on your age and history, I think hormones are most likely, but here's what we can do to be sure."

If the phrase *differential diagnosis* feels too medical, you can get the same result by asking these questions:

- "What else could this be?"
- "What possibilities are you considering?"
- "If it's not this, what else is on the list?"

Scripts You Can Borrow

Sometimes the hardest part of asking good questions is finding the words in the moment, especially when you're anxious, in pain, or trying to process a lot of information quickly. Having a few ready-made phrases can help you stay focused and confident. These aren't magic words, but they give you a starting point to make sure you leave your visit with clarity and a plan.

- "Can you explain that in plain language?"
- "If you were me, what questions would you be asking right now?"
- "What are the worst-case and best-case scenarios here?"
- "What will you be ruling out with this test?"
- "How will I know if I should come back sooner?"

Reflection Prompts

- Think of a past visit: what's a question I wish I had asked, and how could I phrase it now?

- Do I usually ask yes/no questions? How could I reframe one into an open-ended version?

- What kind of answers help me feel confident? Specific numbers, plain-language explanations, or clear next steps?

- How comfortable am I with asking follow-up questions if I don't understand something the first time?

- What's one question I want to make sure I ask at my next visit, no matter what?

Worksheet: My Questions for This Visit

My top concern:

_____

Questions I want to ask *(phrased to invite clear, detailed answers):*

1. _____
   _____

2. _____
   _____

3. _____
   _____

4. _____
   _____

Practice exercise:

Take one yes/no question you might usually ask and rewrite it as an open-ended version.

- Yes/no version: _____

  _____
  _____
  _____
  _____

- Open-ended version: _____

  _____
  _____
  _____
  _____

Skill 7

Bringing Someone with You (or Not)

Walking into an exam room can feel very different when you're not alone. For some people, having a support person by their side makes it easier to speak up, remember details, or feel safe. For others, bringing someone along feels overwhelming, distracting, or simply unnecessary.

The truth is: there's no right answer. What matters is making a choice that supports *you*. This tool helps you think through whether to bring someone, how to prepare them if you do, and how to set boundaries if you'd rather go solo.

Why You Might Want a Support Person

A support person can play many roles during a medical visit. Think about whether any of these resonate with you:

- **Note-taking and memory support.** It can be hard to absorb information in the moment, especially if you're nervous. A support person can write down instructions or test results so you don't have to rely on memory later.
- **Advocacy when you feel dismissed.** If you tend to freeze or get shut down when your concerns aren't taken seriously, a trusted companion can step in and reinforce what you've said.

- **Extra set of ears.** When a visit involves complicated or technical information—like lab results, treatment options, or surgical planning—it helps to have someone else listening who may catch details you miss.
- **Emotional presence.** Medical visits can feel vulnerable. Having someone there to provide reassurance or simply sit with you during a difficult exam can lessen the emotional weight.
- **Practical support.** After sedation, anesthesia, or certain procedures, you may need someone to drive you home or stay with you afterward.

Why You Might Prefer to Go Alone

However, being solo can sometimes make for a stronger or more comfortable visit. Consider whether these issues apply to you:

- **Privacy for sensitive topics.** If you want to talk openly about sexual health, fertility, trauma, or mental health, you may feel freer without someone else in the room.
- **Space for honesty.** Sometimes the presence of a partner, parent, or friend can cause you to edit yourself—or can make a provider edit what they say. Going alone ensures the conversation is direct.
- **Less distraction.** A visit can be harder to manage if you're worried about your support person's reactions, questions, or comfort level.
- **Independence.** Some people simply prefer to handle medical visits on their own, seeing it as part of taking ownership of their health.

Scripts and Strategies for Support

Whether you choose to bring someone with you or go alone, the key is being intentional. If you want company, decide what kind of support would be most useful and communicate that clearly. If you'd rather go solo, set boundaries in a way that's firm but respectful. **Inviting someone in.** If you'd like someone with you, try:

- "Would you come with me to this appointment? It would help me feel supported."
- "I'd like you to be there, but mostly to listen and take notes so I don't miss anything."

Setting boundaries if you prefer to go alone. Privacy is also powerful. If you know you'll do better on your own, you can say,

- "I really appreciate the offer, but I think I want to handle this one on my own."
- "I'll fill you in afterward—I just know I'll be more comfortable solo."

Preparing a Support Person

If you decide to bring someone, set expectations before the visit. Let them know exactly how you'd like them to show up. You are the patient, and you set the tone. The most helpful companions understand their role and stay within it. Clarity up front helps prevent confusion in the exam room and ensures their presence makes the visit easier, not harder. Examples of roles you might assign:

- **Note-taker.** "Can you jot down what the provider says so I can focus on the conversation?"
- **Advocate.** "If I get flustered, can you remind me to ask about ___?"
- **Moral support.** "I don't need you to talk, just being there will help me feel calmer."

Reflection Prompts

- Do I feel more at ease speaking honestly with someone in the room, or do I tend to share more openly when I'm on my own?

- If I bring a support person, what role would be most helpful for me in this visit: taking notes, advocating if I'm dismissed, offering emotional support, or something else?

- What boundaries do I want to set ahead of time about what will or won't be discussed in front of them?

- If I choose to go alone, how will I make sure I still capture the details I need (notes, recording, written summary after the visit)?

Worksheet: My Support Plan

Do I want to bring someone?
- ☐ Yes
- ☐ No
- ☐ Not sure yet

If yes, who? _____

Role I want them to play *(check any that apply)*:
- ☐ Note-taker
- ☐ Advocate/reminder for my questions
- ☐ Emotional support
- ☐ Driver/transportation
- ☐ Other: _____

What I want to tell them ahead of time:

_____

_____

Boundaries I want to set (with them or with my provider):

_____

_____

_____

For Support People

If you've been asked to come along to a visit, it's because your presence matters. Sometimes your job will be to speak up; other times, it's just to sit quietly and hold space. The most important thing is to follow the lead of the person in the exam chair. They are the patient, and this is their visit.

- Ask them what role they want you to play before the appointment.
- If you take notes, stick to facts so they have a clear record later.
- Step in only if they ask or if you see they're being dismissed and want backup.
- Remember: your presence alone can be powerful.

You'll also see "For Support People" boxes included throughout the scenarios later in this workbook. Each one gives you quick, practical guidance on how to show up in that specific situation.

Skill 8

Outlining Your What-Ifs

Anticipate the Unexpected and Create a Plan Before You Need One

Healthcare doesn't always go the way you expect it to. Sometimes it's a middle-of-the-night cramp that makes you sit straight up in bed, or a discharge that doesn't look right, or a medication side effect that has you second-guessing everything you read on the label.

You can't prepare for every possible scenario. But you *can* plan for the ones that would leave you scared, unsure, or scrambling.

This section helps you do exactly that: identify the handful of what-ifs that actually matter most for your life right now, and turn them into concrete action plans. It's not about anticipating catastrophe. It's about lowering the mental load. So that when something unexpected happens, you don't lose precious time trying to figure out what to do or whom to call.

Why This Exercise Matters

Most of us are told how our care *should* go. Told what's normal, what's typical, what to expect in the best-case scenario.

But very few of us are told what to do if things *don't* go as planned.

When you know your next step before something happens, you take panic out of the equation.

This is your chance to prepare with calm clarity instead of reactive fear.

Think of this as your "if this, then that" plan for your body.

Because being informed doesn't make you paranoid, it makes you powerful.

Step 1: Name Your Top Five What-Ifs

Start by asking yourself, *What are the moments that would feel most stressful, confusing, or overwhelming if they happened tonight?*

To give you an idea, here are examples of what-if questions you may have.

Procedures or Interventions
- What if my IUD pain gets worse overnight?
- What if my bleeding after a biopsy or medication abortion feels heavier than they said it would?
- What if my C-section incision looks red or starts leaking fluid?

Pregnancy and Postpartum
- What if I start having contractions earlier than expected?
- What if my water breaks and I live far from my hospital?
- What if my milk hasn't come in and I'm worried my baby isn't feeding enough?
- What if I feel empty, angry, or disconnected after birth?

Medications or Side Effects
- What if my new birth control is making me depressed or anxious?
- What if I miss a dose? Or accidentally take one twice?
- What if I start a new medication and my period suddenly changes?

Chronic or Unpredictable Symptoms
- What if my pelvic pain flares up and I can't get in to see anyone for days?
- What if I faint or feel dizzy and don't know if it's serious?
- What if my partner notices something wrong before I do? What should they look for?

Access or Logistics

- What if I can't reach my provider after hours?
- What if my pharmacy is closed or out of my medication?
- What if I'm out of town when something happens?

Emotional or Relational Scenarios

- What if I feel dismissed again and freeze up during my next visit?
- What if I start panicking before an exam or procedure?
- What if someone close to me doesn't support my medical decisions?

These aren't hypotheticals, they're real-world possibilities that many people encounter every day.

Use this table to identify yours before you ask your clinician what to do:

What If ...	Why It Worries Me	What I'd Want to Know Ahead of Time
1.		
2.		
3.		
4.		
5.		

Step 2: Turn Each What-If into a Plan

Once you've identified your biggest what-ifs, it's time to bring them up and get your questions answered.

This is where preparation turns into empowerment.

Many people never get to ask these questions because visits move fast. But naming your concerns directly helps your clinician meet you where you are.

You're not being dramatic or overprepared; you're being proactive.

Use this table to organize what you want to ask and what guidance you receive:

What If ...	What to Do	Notes

Step 3: Check In with Yourself

Once you've made your list and talked it through, take a minute to notice how you feel.

Does this exercise make you feel calmer? More aware? Maybe a little nervous at first, but then more grounded?

Write it down.

This process is just as much about emotional reassurance as it is about logistics.

How I Felt Before	How I Feel After	What I Learned About Myself

Step 4: Revisit and Update

Your what-ifs will likely change over time, and that's perfectly normal.

What feels urgent now might not even cross your mind six months from today.

Set a note or reminder to check in with this list every few months, or anytime your care situation changes. New medication? New diagnosis? New stage of life? Another trimester? Update your what-ifs. and go through the process again.

Final Thought

You can't control every outcome.

But you *can* control how prepared you are to respond if things shift unexpectedly.

This is about listening to your nerves and also being ready. It's about having the peace of mind that comes with knowing you've already thought through the hard stuff, and you have a plan in place, just in case.

Because when you already know what to do, the unknown loses some of its power over you.

Skill 9

Reflecting After a Visit

Because clarity doesn't always happen in the room. Walking out of an appointment doesn't mean the visit is over. The truth is, the real work often happens afterward. When you sit in your car, replay the conversation in your head, or scroll back through your notes. Reflection gives you a chance to pause, sort through what actually happened, and decide how you want to use that experience moving forward.

The goal isn't to pick apart every detail or relive the hard parts, it's to translate the visit into clarity. Reflection helps you do the following:

- **Keep what worked.** Even a rushed appointment might hold moments worth remembering: a provider who explained something clearly, a question you asked that landed well, a piece of advice that felt useful.
- **Name what didn't.** Writing down what left you feeling dismissed, confused, or unsafe turns vague frustration into something you can act on.
- **Close the loop.** Visits rarely resolve everything at once. Reflection helps you track unanswered questions, identify follow-up needs, and sketch out your next steps.
- **Strengthen your future self.** Each time you take stock after a visit, you leave breadcrumbs for the next appointment: what to ask, what to avoid, and how you want to show up.

Why It Matters

Reflection isn't just a journaling exercise, it's a strategy for self-advocacy. After a visit, especially with a new provider, your emotions and observations are still fresh. Writing them down captures what your nervous system noticed before time smooths over the details.

That matters because medical encounters are often charged spaces, especially if you're navigating reproductive care, gender-affirming care, or trauma-informed care. In the moment, it's easy to miss red flags or minimize your own instincts. Reflecting afterward helps you separate *how you felt* from *what actually happened*, so you can see patterns and make more informed choices moving forward.

When you reflect after meeting a new provider, you're doing two important things at once:

- **You're assessing fit.** Is this someone who listens? Who explains clearly? Who treats your questions with respect? The notes you take after a first visit become the evidence you'll use to decide whether this is a provider to keep or one to replace.
- **You're building continuity for yourself.** The medical system isn't designed to remember your story from visit to visit, but you can. Reflection helps you create your own throughline, so you don't have to start from scratch every time.

It's also about reclaiming power. In a system that often makes patients feel rushed or powerless, slowing down afterward is a quiet act of resistance. It says, "I deserve to understand what just happened. I deserve to make meaning of my care. I deserve to carry my story forward on my own terms."

Think of this as a skill you practice, not once, but every time. After each visit, you're not just closing a chapter; you're writing the next one with more clarity, confidence, and control.

Step 1: What Was Discussed

Start by grounding yourself in the facts. What actually happened in the room?
    Write down anything that stands out before it fades.

- What did I clearly explain to my provider today? _____
- What did I learn today? _____

- What tests, imaging, or exams did they recommend (if any)? _____

- What explanations or diagnoses were offered (if any)? _____

- What's the plan—watch and wait, switch medications, further evaluation, treatment? _____

Step 2: Understanding and Clarity

Use this space to check your understanding of the information shared.

- How well did my provider explain my options? _____

- Do I understand what might be causing my symptoms? _____

- Did I feel pressured toward a specific method or plan? _____

- What questions did I get answered? _____

- What questions do I still have? _____

Step 3: Emotional Check-In

Your emotional experience is part of your medical data. How you *felt* during the visit is as important as what was said.

- What helped me feel in control or supported? _____

- What left me feeling dismissed or unsure? _____

- Did I feel believed and taken seriously? Why or why not? _____

- Was anything dismissed or minimized that I want to revisit later? _____

- How did I feel emotionally after the visit? (Relieved? Frustrated? Exhausted? Validated?) _____

- What do I need—emotionally or practically—to move forward? _____

Quick Check *(check all that apply):*

☐ Heard ☐ Respected ☐ Supported ☐ Rushed
☐ Ignored ☐ Judged ☐ Unsafe ☐ Other: _____

Step 4: What Worked and What Didn't

This is where you make sense of patterns so you can build on what felt right and change what didn't.

What worked:

• What explanations made sense to me? _____

• Was there a clear plan or next step that felt helpful? _____

What didn't:

• Did I leave with more confusion than clarity? _____

• Was I interrupted, rushed, or dismissed? _____

• Did anything feel judgmental, shaming, or unsafe? _____

Step 5: Next Steps and Follow-Up

Turn your reflections into an action plan.

• What are my next concrete steps (tests, referrals, meds, follow-up visits)? _____
_____

• When will I hear about results, and how? _____
_____

• Who should I call if things change or get worse? _____
_____

• Do I feel confident in the next step—or do I want a second opinion? _____
_____

Step 6: Bigger Picture Reflection

Zoom out for perspective. These questions help you connect this visit to your overall care story.

- What did I learn about my provider? Their style, their strengths, or their limits?
  _____
  _____

- What did I learn about myself as a patient? How I ask questions, how I advocate, or what I need to feel supported? _____
  _____

- If a friend described this same visit to me, what advice would I give them? _____
  _____
  _____

- What's most concerning to me right now? _____
  _____

- What would feel like success in addressing this? _____
  _____

- How is this affecting my relationship with my body? _____
  _____

- What kind of support would help me feel more confident? _____
  _____

Step 7: Notes for Future You

This is your space to leave yourself a message—what to remember, avoid, or carry forward.

- Next time, I want to ask about: _____

- If I feel dismissed, I will try this script: _____

- Next time, I want to bring (support person, notes, checklist, etc.): _____

Key Takeaway

Healthcare can feel rushed, impersonal, or out of your control. Reflection slows things down. It's where you turn reaction into understanding and uncertainty into direction. Writing down what worked, what didn't, and what comes next helps you rebuild trust, both in your care and in yourself. This isn't just about remembering details. It's about reclaiming your story in a system that too often leaves patients out of their own narrative.

Skill 10

When Care Doesn't Go Right: Speaking Up, Salvaging, and Knowing When to Leave

No one expects a medical visit to go badly. But sometimes it does.

It might be subtle. A rushed answer. A dismissive comment. A provider who seems distracted. Or it might be more serious and leave you feeling unheard, disrespected, or unsafe. When this happens, it can feel like you're trapped. You've already waited weeks (sometimes months) for the appointment, rearranged work, lined up childcare, driven across town. Walking out feels impossible.

But you do have choices. Sometimes you can salvage a visit by speaking up in the moment. Other times, reflection afterward will tell you whether this relationship can be repaired or whether it's time to move on. And if changing clinicians isn't possible, you still have strategies to protect yourself and press for better care.

Step 1: Course Correct When Needed

Not every misstep means the relationship is over. Providers get rushed, distracted, or simply miss signals. Speaking up gives them a chance to correct course—and gives you the chance to get what you came for.

Scripts to try:

- If the conversation feels rushed: "I know time is tight, but I need to make sure we cover this today."
- If you're brushed off with "that's normal": "It doesn't feel normal for me. Can you explain why you think that?"
- If you're redirected too soon: "Before we move on, I'd like to finish talking through this."
- If the tone feels judgmental: "I'd like to focus on solutions that work for me, not just what I 'should' be doing."
- If you need clarity: "What else could this be? Can you walk me through your differential diagnoses?"

Step 2: If a Visit Is Still Bad

Sometimes, no matter what you try, the visit doesn't recover. When that happens, you still have options.

In the moment:

- **Acknowledge and pivot.** "I don't feel like my concern is being addressed. Can we go back to it?"
- **Name the mismatch.** "If this isn't the right visit to cover this, what's the best way to get the time I need?"

After the visit:

Take time to reflect. Bad visits are draining and can shake your trust, but reflection turns frustration into clarity. Ask yourself,

- "Did I feel heard and respected?"
- "Did I leave with answers? Or at least a plan?"
- "Was this a one-time misstep, or a repeated pattern?"
- "Do I feel comfortable giving them another chance?"

Step 3: Knowing When to Walk Away

Leaving a provider can be hard. Insurance, waitlists, logistics all make it complicated. But you don't owe loyalty to a relationship that isn't working. Walking away is not "being difficult." It is advocating for the care you deserve.

Signs that it may be time to leave:

- You regularly feel dismissed or not believed.
- Pain, bleeding, or symptoms are minimized without explanation.
- You hear judgmental or shaming comments.
- Your identity (race, gender, weight, sexuality, disability) is treated as the problem.
- You leave feeling worse about yourself than when you arrived.
- You feel unsafe, disrespected, or ignored.

Step 4: Finding a New Clinician

Starting over can feel daunting, but you're not starting from scratch. You now know what didn't work, which gives you a clearer idea of what you need.

Where to look:

- Ask trusted friends, family, or community networks.
- Search directories for providers who highlight inclusivity, trauma-informed care, or LGBTQ+/BIPOC-centered practices.
- Use your insurance database (but double-check reviews).
- If you feel comfortable, ask your current provider for a referral. They may know who's a better fit.

What to ask when you call:

- "Does this provider see patients with [my concern] regularly?"
- "Do they have experience working with [identity or condition that matters to me]?"
- "What's the average wait time for an appointment?"

What to watch for early on:

- Were you treated respectfully at check-in or on the phone?
- Did the provider listen without interrupting?
- Did they explain things in language that made sense?
- Did you leave feeling listened to or shut down?

Step 5: If Changing Isn't Possible

Sometimes switching isn't an option because of geography, insurance, or limited providers. In those cases, you still deserve tools to protect yourself.

If switching really isn't possible:

- **Document everything.** Keep detailed notes, request visit summaries, save portal messages.
- **Apply external pressure.** Contact your insurance, file a complaint with the state medical board, or connect with advocacy organizations.
- **Find workarounds.** Ask if you can see another clinician in the practice. Perhaps you may want to see an advanced practice provider like a nurse practitioner or a physician associate. Explore family medicine, internal medicine, urgent care, or telehealth for certain needs.

Scripts when you're not getting the care you need:

- "If this isn't your area of expertise, can you refer me to someone who specializes in it?"
- "I'm documenting that I requested [test/treatment] and was declined. Please note your reasoning in my chart."
- "I understand you don't want to pursue this. Can you explain your reasoning so I can understand your decision?"
- "Since we disagree, I'd like a second opinion. Can you facilitate that?"

Escalation strategies within a system if needed:

- Ask for refusals to be documented in your chart with the provider's name and date.
- Request to speak with a supervising physician, department head, or patient advocate.
- File a formal complaint about your care.

Long-term strategies:

- Build relationships with additional access points (urgent care, telehealth, family medicine).
- Connect with patient communities for peer support and provider recommendations.
- Keep meticulous records so you're always prepared to advocate effectively with new providers when opportunities arise.

Reflection Prompts

- What parts of my last visit felt supportive? What felt harmful?

- Did I leave with clarity and a plan or just more confusion?

- If a friend described this visit to me, what advice would I give them?

- Do I feel comfortable giving this provider another chance, or is my energy better spent finding someone new?

- Are there any additional qualities I want in a provider that were missing last time?

- If I can't leave this provider now, what's one step I can take to protect myself and keep the door open for better care later?

Key Takeaway

Bad visits happen. What matters isn't pretending they didn't, but deciding what you do next. Sometimes that means speaking up and trying to shift the moment. Sometimes it means taking time to process and giving it another chance. And sometimes it means walking away and finding care that fits better.

The important thing is this: you get to decide.

Part Two

REAL-LIFE SCENARIOS AND SUPPORT

Because reproductive healthcare isn't theoretical; sometimes you need the words before you walk into the room

Now that you've built your foundation, it's time to take it into the real world. From here on out, this book shifts from reading material to real-life workbook. These pages are for you—to mark up, reflect in, and return to. Use them as a journal. Scribble in the margins. Highlight what hits. Dog-ear the pages you'll want to revisit.

Pick what works for you. Each scenario stands on its own. So start wherever you are. Maybe you're bringing your teen to their first OB-GYN visit. Maybe you're navigating fertility as a same-sex couple, asking for pain management, or figuring out how to talk about menopause with a provider who keeps brushing you off. Wherever you are, my hope is that there is a guide here to meet you.

Not everything in these pages will apply to you. Maybe it'll help a friend, a sister, a daughter, a patient. Share these pages wide and far. Rip them out if you want. Send pictures. This information is meant to move. I want it out in the world, helping whoever needs it.

That's how change happens. When one of us learns how to advocate, it opens the door a little wider for everyone else.

These aren't hypotheticals. They're real, lived-in, messy, beautiful moments people face every day. Often without a map. Each scenario walks you through what to expect, what to ask, what to watch for, and what to say when things go sideways.

This section builds on everything that came before it: all the groundwork, all the skills, and all the confidence you've been building. Now it's about putting those skills in motion.

These pages are your prep. Your permission slip. Your steady hand before you walk into a vulnerable room. Because even if the system feels impossible, you still have options. You still have power. And you still deserve care that sees you.

There's no way to cover every corner of reproductive medicine in one workbook. These scenarios center on gynecological care, with some coverage of fertility and abortion, but they stop short of full obstetrical care. That's because pregnancy, labor, and postpartum care deserve their own depth and their own dedicated space. This workbook was never meant to be a comprehensive medical encyclopedia. It's meant to be a practical, emotional, and deeply human guide for the places people most often fall through the cracks.

These scenarios were chosen because they represent the most common, and the most misunderstood, encounters in reproductive healthcare. The moments where people are most likely to feel dismissed, unprepared, or alone. Annual exams that turn awkward or invasive. Birth control conversations that turn judgmental. Menstrual or pelvic pain that gets brushed off. Fertility appointments where hope and fear live side by side. Abortion care that's met with stigma instead of support. These are the visits that shape how people feel about their bodies, their autonomy, and their place in the medical system.

Gynecology sits at the intersection of gender, medicine, and power. It's one of the first places many people learn what it feels like to be believed. Or not. To be respected. Or not. It's where the trust between patients and medicine is often built, broken, or rebuilt again. And because gynecology touches everything from contraception to menopause, it's also one of the most consistent, recurring relationships people have with healthcare throughout their lives.

By focusing here, we get to practice skills that matter everywhere: asking better questions, setting boundaries, and navigating bias in real time. When you can advocate for yourself during a pelvic exam or after a miscarriage, you build muscles you can carry into every other corner of medicine, whether that's a mammogram, a cardiology consult, or your child's pediatrician appointment.

The power is in the nuance. In slowing down, zooming in, and looking closely at the moments that medicine often rushes past. The point isn't to overwhelm you with every possible scenario. It's to meet you in the most common and least supported ones, and to show you how preparation, language, and trust can change the entire experience.

Because the truth is, when you start to understand what's broken in gynecology, you start to see what's broken across the whole system. And when you learn how to advocate in these rooms, the most personal, most intimate rooms, you learn how to advocate anywhere.

That's why we start here. Not because it's the only place where change is needed, but because it's the place where change can start.

FOUNDATIONS OF CARE AND IDENTITY-BASED NAVIGATION

Scenario 1

Bringing Your Teen In for Their First Visit

How to model trust, support privacy, and set your teen up for a lifetime of empowered care

This visit isn't just about reproductive health. It's also about teaching self-advocacy.

This is their visit. Not yours.

You're here to model trust and support. Not to take over.

The goal? Help your teen build confidence, feel safe in medical spaces, and begin developing good patient habits. You don't need to control the visit. In fact, you shouldn't. You can prepare them to lead it. You can prepare them to be their own health advocate from a young age.

Before you walk into the room, talk to your teen. Ask them what *they* want to get out of the visit. Their needs are what matter most. Let them know they'll be taking the lead. You're just there as backup.

You can say, "This visit is yours. You get to ask the questions, skip anything that doesn't feel right, and tell the provider what you need. I'm here if you want me, but you're in charge."

And "I'm happy to step out if you want privacy at any point. I trust you completely."

This is the beginning of learning how to speak up, ask questions, and build trust in healthcare spaces. Let them try. Let them lead.

What to Expect

You may have never forgotten your first OB-GYN visit.

Maybe it was awkward. Maybe it was confusing. Maybe it was a blur of paper gowns, cold instruments, and someone asking you if you were sexually active before you even understood the question. For many people, that first appointment set the tone for how they'd think about reproductive healthcare for years, sometimes decades.

But here's the good news: it's different now.

That old-school approach is no longer the standard. For most teens, the first OB-GYN visit doesn't involve a pelvic exam. In fact, if you've scheduled just a routine visit or birth control consult they'll usually keep their clothes on. It's not about stirrups, it's about starting a relationship. Most first visits are just a conversation. A chance to talk about periods, puberty, consent, birth control, and what to expect as their body changes. And now, most individuals won't need a Pap smear or pelvic exam until age 21. So you can tell your teen to take a deep breath.

The provider should speak directly to your teen, invite their input, and explain their rights clearly. They should make space for your teen to ask questions in an environment free of judgment, pressure, or awkward silence. And if that's not happening? You can advocate for it.

Most providers trained in adolescent care will ask to speak with your teen privately for part of the visit. That's a good thing. It gives your teen a safe space to ask questions and advocate for themselves, without worrying about your reaction. But if the provider doesn't offer that, you can prompt it toward the end of the visit if it feels right or needed:

"Would you like to have a few minutes alone with them? I'm happy to step out."

If your teen has symptoms like increased discharge, pain, or difficulty inserting a tampon, a pelvic exam may be recommended. But it should never be automatic, rushed, or done without a clear explanation and consent.

Your teen has the right to ask these questions:

"Can you explain what you're doing and why?"
"I'm nervous. Can we go slowly?"
"Actually, I'd rather not do this today."

And don't forget the ride home. Debrief gently. Not with interrogation, but with care. Try:

"How did that feel?"
"Was anything confusing or surprising?"
"Would you want to go back to that provider again?"

Let them lead. Let them feel in charge. This visit doesn't have to cover everything. It just needs to be a start. One that shows them their body isn't something to fear or be ashamed of, and that healthcare can be a place of safety and empowerment.

You're not just helping your teen get care. You're helping them learn how to advocate for their needs. Teaching them that that their voice and their needs should be centered in the room.

That's the beginning of trust.
That's the beginning of agency.
That's what they deserve.

Pre-Visit Planning

This is made to help you and your teen prepare for the appointment. Made to ensure you both know what the goals of the visit are. I recommend that you go through it with your teen or share it with them if that's more comfortable.

What are the goals for this visit? *(check all that apply)*

☐ Get to know the provider
☐ Talk about options for management of menses or body changes
☐ Ask about birth control for pregnancy prevention or any additional reason
☐ Ask about pain or symptoms that are bothersome
☐ Discuss sexually transmitted infection testing or protection
☐ Talk about gender, orientation, or identity
☐ Something else: _____

What are some questions you or your teen might want to ask?

_____

_____

Pertinent prior history worth sharing:

_____

_____

What concerns or worries are coming up?

Your teen's concerns:

_____

Your concerns as a parent or caregiver:

_____

Anything else that might help the visit go better?

Any particular care needs? Sensory needs?

Does your teen want you in the visit or sitting in the waiting room?

_____

_____

Scenario 2

Being Overweight in the Exam Room

How to redirect bias, ask for inclusive care, and be treated as a patient—not a project

---

A Note on Language: "Overweight" Versus "Fat"

Language matters—especially when it's used to talk about your body.

You may notice this book uses both *overweight* and *fat* in different places. That's intentional.

- *Overweight* is often the term used in medical records and clinical conversations.
- *Fat* is a word many body positive individuals are reclaiming—using it as a neutral or empowering identity, not an insult.

Fat isn't a diagnosis. It's a descriptor. It's not something to apologize for. And for many, it feels more honest and less pathologizing than *overweight*.

You are not obligated to use either.

Use the language that feels right to you, and reject anything that doesn't.

The Real Story

You walk in for a Pap smear. Or a yeast infection. Or maybe just to establish care.

And somehow, the conversation has shifted. It's no longer about your reason for coming in. It's about your weight.

You didn't bring it up. You didn't ask for advice. But suddenly, the provider is recommending a diet. Suggesting you "get your body mass index (BMI) under control." Telling you that "a lot of these symptoms could improve if you lost some weight."

And just like that, you've gone from *patient* to *project*. Your reason for coming in becomes a side note.

Here's the truth: weight bias is baked into medicine.

It shows up in textbooks, in training, in how exam tables are sized, and in how gowns are stocked.

It shows up in the assumption that your body is the problem before anyone has listened to a word you say.

That doesn't mean every clinician is cruel. It means most were trained to see weight as a diagnosis instead of one small part of a much bigger story.

There's another way. One rooted in respect, curiosity, and care that focuses on behaviors and health. Not body size.

This type of approach doesn't tie your health to the number on a scale. It doesn't assume thin automatically means healthy or fat automatically means sick. It centers dignity, real listening, and individualized care.

You deserve that kind of care. You deserve to be treated like a whole person, not a BMI. And you deserve to not have every damn conversation circle back to your weight.

Even if your provider believes weight *may* play a role in your symptoms, they owe you more than "Just lose weight." That's not a treatment plan. That's a brush-off. And that's what gets people dismissed, undiagnosed, and harmed.

If you've ever delayed care to avoid being weighed. If you've searched for answers on your own because past visits left you feeling dismissed. If you've tried to change your body just to feel safer walking into an exam room. You're not overreacting. You're responding to a system that taught you your value is related to a number on the scale. A system that made you believe your body had to earn care.

You Deserve Better

If the provider doesn't listen, if they dismiss your concerns or attribute everything to your size without investigating further, you are allowed to walk out.

Yes, finding affirming providers takes effort. But they *do* exist.

You can ask when booking:

- "Does this provider use a weight-inclusive approach rather than focusing solely on weight loss?"
- "Are the exam tables, equipment, and gowns accessible for larger-bodied patients?"

And if they hesitate, that tells you a lot.

Your body is not the barrier to care. *Bias is.* You deserve to walk into an exam room and feel safe. Seen. Respected.

You are allowed to say the following:

- "I'm not here to talk about my weight today."
- "Please focus on the concern I came in for."
- "If you don't think my body size is causing this, let's move on."
- "Would your recommendations be the same for someone in a smaller body with this exact concern?"

You are allowed to do the following:

- Ask for accommodations, such as a gown that fits, a larger blood pressure cuff, an exam table that appropriately supports your body, or a different sized speculum that has worked better for your anatomy in the past.
- Say, "Please note in my chart that I decline to be weighed unless it's medically necessary." Or "I'd like to be weighed standing backward. You can document my weight in the chart but I don't want to hear it said out loud."
- Bring someone with you to back you up, take notes, or redirect the conversation.
- Expect respect, not judgment.

Identity Check-In: What Language Feels Right to Me?

When I describe my body to others, I typically say:

_____

_____

Words that feel neutral or affirming to me:

_____

Words that feel medicalized, shaming, stigmatizing, triggering, or hurtful:

_____

I want my provider to use these terms when discussing my body:

_____

And I want them to avoid these terms:

_____

Pre-Visit Planning

My goal for this visit is as follows:

_____

_____

What I want to ask or clarify:
"Are my symptoms being fully evaluated, or just attributed to weight?"
"Can we discuss risk without judgment?"
"What equipment or accommodations are available for my body?"

Accommodations I may want to ask for:
☐ Gown in my size
☐ Larger blood pressure cuff
☐ Different sized speculums if needed
☐ Exam table that supports higher weight
☐ Option to skip the scale unless medically necessary

For Support People

They've likely internalized years of shame about their body and may expect medical appointments to be full of judgment rather than care. They need someone who sees their worth beyond their weight and refuses to let bias masquerade as medical advice.

Rebuilding trust. Remind them that their health concerns are valid regardless of their size. Help them recognize that biased treatment says nothing about their worth and everything about the provider's limitations.

Provider shopping. Help them find practitioners who practice weight-inclusive care. Celebrate providers who treat them with dignity and see them as a whole person.

Processing experiences. After difficult appointments, help them separate their legitimate health concerns from any shame imposed by biased providers.

If you're joining for the visit. Don't let weight become the scapegoat for every symptom. You might need to redirect: "Let's focus on what's actually happening with their body today."

Scenario 3

Trans, Nonbinary, and Intersex Gynecologic Care

What affirming care actually looks like, how to set boundaries, and what you can ask for before and during the visit

This scenario was reviewed in collaboration with **Delia Sosa** (they/them). At the time of writing, Delia is a fourth-year medical student and aspiring OB-GYN whose work focuses on advancing affirming, inclusive care for LGBTQ+, intersex, and gender-diverse patients. Delia serves as the executive director of the Medical Student Pride Alliance (MSPA), a national organization empowering queer and trans medical students to lead with equity and compassion in medicine.

Delia reviewed, edited, and helped shape this section to ensure it reflects both the science and the lived realities of trans, nonbinary, and intersex people navigating OB-GYN care. Their insight, expertise, and commitment to inclusive medicine brought depth, clarity, and authenticity to every word.

This Isn't "Women's Health," It's Your Health

If you've ever felt like you don't belong in obstetric and gynecologic spaces, you're not imagining it. The system wasn't built with you in mind. Maybe it's that there's only a *Women's Health* magazine that sits on the table, perhaps the forms ask "sex: male or female," or someone calls your deadname aloud.

It's not always loud. It's not always violent. It may not be intentional. But sometimes it's enough to make you feel like your body is too complicated. Like your identity is an inconvenience. And you should never have to feel this way.

Your care doesn't have to fit someone else's labels. But it is necessary, valid, and lifesaving. This isn't about opting into "women's health." It's about getting care that fits your anatomy, symptoms, and needs—without having to defend your identity in the process.

You're not asking for special treatment. You're not asking them to reinvent the wheel. You're asking for real care. And you deserve it.

When someone misgenders you, skips over your concerns, or forces a conversation you didn't ask for, it can be hard to speak up in the moment. You shouldn't have to correct your provider just to feel safe. You shouldn't have to educate the room you came to for care.

This section of the workbook is here to help you navigate those moments by outlining what affirming care should look and feel like before you walk in and while you're in the room, along with ways to redirect the visit if things go off track. You'll find scripts, questions, and strategies to help you stay in control, whether you're there for a wellness visit, a birth control consult, a prenatal visit, or something else.

Your identity is not up for debate. And you have the right to access care that acknowledges and addresses you and your needs.

Intersex Care Matters, Too

Intersex people are often erased from conversations about both gender and healthcare, even in spaces that claim to be inclusive. But intersex variations are a natural part of human diversity, and intersex patients deserve care that honors that reality.

If you were born with an intersex variation, or learned later on in adolescence or adulthood that you have an intersex variation, you may have experienced unnecessary surgeries, hormone interventions, or invasive exams early in life. Often without your consent. That history can make medical spaces and especially reproductive health spaces especially fraught. You deserve trauma-informed, consent-based care that centers your autonomy and comfort, not assumptions about what your body "should" look like or do.

Affirming intersex care means your provider does the following:

- Understands that "normalizing" surgeries are a form of bodily harm when done without informed consent
- Uses language that aligns with your lived experience, not outdated or pathologizing terms
- Focuses on your current health and comfort, not on "correcting" or making a spectacle of anatomy
- Respects that your medical history is yours to share (or not share) on your terms
- Acknowledges long-term implications of certain intersex variations and the early management of them and how to address those implications (e.g., osteoporosis if ovaries/testes/gonads were removed prematurely)

You're allowed to say:

- "I have an intersex variation and want to make sure this visit is handled respectfully and without assumptions."
- "I'd like to discuss my care without focusing on past surgeries or anatomy unless it's relevant to today's visit."
- "Can we go over what exams are actually necessary and why?"
- "Have you treated patients with my intersex variation before?"

Intersex care isn't a footnote. It's part of the broader fight for bodily autonomy and informed consent. Your body is not a medical mystery. It's your home. You deserve care that treats it, and you, with respect.

Before You Walk In

An affirming clinic will do the following:

- Include space for chosen name and pronouns on intake forms
- Use gender-inclusive language from staff to provider

- Be up front about whether they've received LGBTQIA+ competency training
- Understand that obstetric and gynecologic care isn't just for cisgender women

You are absolutely allowed to call ahead and ask questions such as these:

- "I'm a trans/nonbinary/intersex. Does this provider have experience with gender-inclusive obstetrics/gynecology?"
- "Do you have any testimonials from trans or nonbinary patients who have been to your clinic before?"
- "Can you confirm that my name and pronouns will be used correctly at check-in and during the visit?"
- "Has the staff received LGBTQIA+ cultural competency training?"
- "I'd feel more comfortable waiting in my car than in the waiting room. Is that an option?"

If You're in the Room

You are allowed to be clear about what you need.

- "I've had bad experiences before. I need this visit to be intentional and respectful."
- "Please use my correct pronouns and chosen name, even if the chart says otherwise."
- "I'd like you to walk me through everything you're doing, before you do it."

If they mess up? You can correct them. You are not making it awkward. You are asking to be treated with dignity.

If you're there for care that includes a pelvic exam, you deserve consent-based, trauma-informed, gender-affirming care. Full stop. Every time.

You can say:

- "I want to skip the exam today. I just want to talk. If I feel comfortable, can I come back another day if it's needed?"
- "I'd prefer to stay dressed until it's time for the physical exam."
- "Please walk me through every step, starting from before you touch me."

This is not too much to ask. This is the bare minimum for safety, dignity, and respect.

Tips: Navigating the Visit

- Bring a support person, if that feels safe.
- Write down your questions or scripts ahead of time.
- Let the provider know what language feels comfortable for your anatomy.
- You can request a provider of a specific gender if that helps you feel safer.

Start Where You Are

It's important to be clear about what you're going in for and to understand the scope of what your visit can actually cover. One visit can't do everything. And that's okay.

If you've avoided the doctor for years because of past trauma, dysphoria, discrimination, or just not knowing where to start, you're not alone. You haven't failed. You're not behind.

You can start from wherever you are. Whether that means scheduling your first visit in years, going in only to talk (not for an exam), or asking questions to test how safe a provider feels, every step counts. Rebuilding trust in your care doesn't happen overnight. It happens one visit, one boundary, one honest moment at a time.

Disclosing Hormone or Surgical History

You don't have to share anything you're not comfortable sharing. But if you feel safe, letting your provider know about past surgeries and/or hormone use can help them offer more accurate, personalized care. Your provider should meet that information with care and professionalism, not judgment. Sharing your history isn't about defending your identity, it's about making sure your care fits *you*.

Preventive Care Matters

Your anatomy still needs care. Even if you no longer identify with the labels it's usually given.

If you have a cervix, you still need Pap smears to screen for cervical cancer. Even if you're on testosterone or haven't had a period in years. If exams are triggering, painful, or dysphoric, you're allowed to ask for alternatives or adjustments. You can say: "Are there options for Pap smears that respect my comfort and boundaries?" or "Can we go slowly and narrate the steps together?" There are providers who will listen and adapt. There is also an option to do a human papillomavirus (HPV) self-swab, which would be followed by a Pap smear only if the result is positive.

If you have breast tissue, even after top surgery, you may still need mammograms or chest imaging depending on how much tissue remains and your personal or family risk. Risk is based on remaining tissue, not gender.

If you have a uterus or ovaries, you're still at risk for conditions like fibroids, endometriosis, ovarian cysts, or cancer. If you're experiencing pelvic pain, irregular bleeding, or unexplained gastrointestinal symptoms, you deserve to be taken seriously.

Testosterone can also cause the vaginal and cervical tissue to thin, making exams more uncomfortable or painful for some people. That's not your fault. Your provider should be trauma-informed, gentle, and slow. You're allowed to ask for breaks, explain your boundaries, and expect consent every step of the way. You can also ask for a smaller speculum to be used if that is more comfortable for you.

Preventive care isn't about gender. It's about safety, anatomy, and your right to be cared for without shame.

What About Pregnancy?

It's a common misconception that testosterone works as birth control—but it doesn't.

Even if you haven't had a period in months, or years, you can still get pregnant while on testosterone. That's because ovulation doesn't always stop entirely, and it can return unexpectedly, especially if your testosterone dose changes or isn't consistent. Many people have conceived while on testosterone, often without realizing ovulation had occurred.

If you're having sex with someone who can get you pregnant, it's important to talk about contraception. Even if you're not bleeding regularly or if pregnancy feels emotionally distant or dysphoric. You have every right to protect your body in a way that respects your identity and your goals. That doesn't mean going on estrogen-heavy pills or submitting to methods that feel wrong for you. It means exploring what fits.

You have options:

- **A hormonal or nonhormonal intrauterine device (IUD),** which provides long-term, reversible protection—some of which can also reduce or eliminate bleeding.

- **Barrier methods,** like condoms or internal condoms, which are hormone-free and can be used on your own terms.
- **Progesterone only options:** The shot (Depo-Provera), the Nexplanon arm implant, or progestin-only birth control pills, which may align with your goals if you're looking to avoid estrogen. (Hormonal IUDs are also progesterone only.)
- And if you're looking for something permanent, you can also ask about **sterilization options**, such as a hysterectomy or bilateral salpingectomy (removal of the fallopian tubes that carry an egg from the ovaries to the uterus) that don't require hormone involvement at all.

You're allowed to say:

- "I'm on testosterone, but I know that doesn't prevent pregnancy. What are my options that won't interfere with my hormones or dysphoria?"
- "I want pregnancy protection and bleeding control, but I don't want estrogen. What would be a good choice for me?"
- "I need contraception that's both effective and gender-affirming. Can we talk through my options?"

There is no one right way to manage pregnancy risk, only what feels safe and right for *you*. Your provider should never assume what kind of sex you're having or what risks are relevant. That's their job to ask respectfully, not your job to educate or over-explain. You deserve options that protect your safety *and* affirm your identity.

Body-Based Care: Options for Comfort and Control

Hormonal IUDs can be a powerful option for managing bleeding, especially if you're looking to reduce or stop your period altogether. They release progestin locally within the uterus rather than systemically throughout the body, and contain no estrogen. This makes them a good fit for many trans and nonbinary patients who want to suppress bleeding without disrupting testosterone therapy.

In addition to helping with bleeding and dysphoria, a hormonal IUD is also one of the most effective forms of reversible birth control. IUDs provide long-term protection with the option to remove it anytime. It can ease menstrual pain, lighten or stop periods, and help make pelvic care more comfortable and predictable.

Topical estrogen is commonly used for symptoms like vaginal dryness, tearing, or discomfort—whether or not you're on testosterone. It comes in several forms, including vaginal creams, tablets, or rings. I know it may feel counterintuitive to your goals, but, unlike systemic estrogen, this low-dose version acts locally on the tissue, meaning it doesn't affect your overall hormone levels or interfere with testosterone. For many people, topical estrogen improves comfort, tissue elasticity, and sexual function—without compromising identity or goals.

Pelvic floor therapy (PT) can help with pain, tightness, or discomfort during pelvic exams, sex, or following surgery. It's especially beneficial for those who've experienced trauma, medical avoidance, or dysphoria related to pelvic care. You can ask your provider for a trauma-informed or gender-affirming physical therapy referral. And just to be clear, pelvic floor therapy isn't only for postpartum cis women. It's for anyone with a pelvis and pain, and it can be a critical part of affirming, whole-body care.

Questions You're Allowed to Ask

You are *always* allowed to ask questions. You don't need the "right words" to advocate for yourself. You can try these:

- "What birth control options are effective for managing bleeding without estrogen?"
- "Can an IUD help reduce or stop my period? Would that help with my dysphoria?"
- "Does this method interact with testosterone or other hormones I'm taking?"
- "Are there noncontraceptive reasons to consider hormonal care—like acne, pain, or mood?"
- "Can we talk about what symptom relief might look like for dysphoria or dryness?"
- "Are there trans-affirming resources or support groups you can refer me to?"
- "Could pelvic floor therapy help with pain or tightness during exams or sex?"
- "What do I need to consider for pregnancy prevention given my intersex variation?"
- "If I want to participate in a pregnancy with my intersex variation, what are my options?"

Pre-Visit Planning

What I want from this visit:

What I want to ask or learn more about:

☐ Does this provider have experience with gender-affirming care and/or intersex care?
☐ How can I receive care that supports my identity and boundaries?
☐ What are my options if I don't feel safe or respected in the visit?
☐ Can we explore care that's not centered on reproductive assumptions?

What's most important for the provider to understand about me:

Which services I might be discussing today *(check all that apply):*

☐ Annual wellness visit/physical (keep in mind that this is preventative, so you'll likely need another appointment if you're wanting to address other concerns beyond basic needs as well)
☐ Sexually transmitted infection screening
☐ Contraceptive options
☐ Hormonal care
☐ Pain, bleeding, or cycle concerns
☐ Fertility or family-building support
☐ Gender-affirming discussion
☐ Other: _____

What I want to say up front *(feel free to modify or write your own):*

- "I use _____ pronouns. Please use them throughout this visit and in my chart."
- "I've had negative experiences before and want to feel safe here.
- "Please narrate the exam step-by-step."
- "I may need to pause the visit if I start to feel overwhelmed."
- "Let's just talk today—no exam unless I feel ready."

Optional Journal Prompts: Before the Visit

Use these to ground yourself and clarify your needs before your appointment:

- When have I felt most affirmed in a medical setting, and what made it feel that way?

- What boundaries or preferences do I want to hold during this visit?

- What helps me feel safer during vulnerable conversations or exams?

- What red flags am I watching for—and what's my plan if they show up?

Affirming My Identity, Language, and Needs in Care

How I identify:

☐ Trans man   ☐ Trans woman   ☐ Nonbinary   ☐ Genderfluid   ☐ Agender
☐ Queer   ☐ Intersex   ☐ Genderqueer   ☐ Still figuring it out
☐ Prefer not to label   ☐ Other: _____

Language that feels right when talking about my care *(check any)*:

☐ Trans health   ☐ Gynecologic care   ☐ Reproductive health
☐ Pelvic care   ☐ Wellness visit   ☐ Queer-inclusive care   ☐ Intersex care
☐ Other: _____

Words I use for my body:

- Chest/breasts _____
- Genitals/anatomy _____
- Other terms I'd like used: _____

Please avoid these words during the visit:

- _____
- _____

How I want to feel walking in:

☐ Respected   ☐ Seen   ☐ Safe   ☐ In control
☐ Free to ask questions   ☐ Not treated like a stranger in the room
☐ Other: _____

How I want to feel walking out:

☐ Heard   ☐ Affirmed   ☐ Informed   ☐ Ready to return
☐ Like I wasn't misgendered   ☐ Like I didn't have to explain myself
☐ Like my health was prioritized
☐ Other: _____

Communicating with my provider (optional scripts):

- "I use different language for some body parts—can I share what feels comfortable?"
- "My chart has my legal name, but I go by [name] and use [pronouns]. Please use those during this visit."
- "Can you flag my chart to reflect my pronouns and name for future visits?"
- "Please walk me through everything before touching me. I may need to pause or ask questions."

For Support People

They're navigating healthcare in a body the system wasn't built to care for—often facing ignorance, erasure, or outright hostility. What they need most is someone who affirms their identity without hesitation and doesn't excuse discrimination under the guise of "medical concern."

Validation and preparation. Acknowledge that their caution is earned. If they're anxious about seeking care, it's not paranoia, it's wisdom shaped by real harm.

Building a care team. Help them find providers who see their full humanity, not someone who treats their identity as a complication to manage.

Celebrate affirming care when it happens. When they finally find a provider who gets it, help them recognize that as *good care*, not luck. They deserve that experience every time.

If you're joining them for a visit. Be prepared to interrupt disrespect, correct pronouns, and make it clear—through your presence and your words—that their dignity is nonnegotiable.

Scenario 4

Navigating OB-GYN Care as a Black Woman or Birthing Person

How to prepare, advocate, and demand accountability in a system built to dismiss you

This scenario was written in collaboration with reproductive health advocate and powerhouse **Kaitlyn Joshua**. Kaitlyn is a national leader in reproductive rights advocacy and the cofounder of Abortion in America. She bravely shared her personal experience with miscarriage and the devastating impact of abortion bans in the South on the national stage at the 2024 Democratic National Convention.

As a non-Black clinician, I know this is not my lived experience, and it would have been wrong to write it alone. Kaitlyn reviewed, edited, and helped shape this section to ensure it reflects the lived realities of Black women and birthing people navigating reproductive care in America.

Before You Walk In

Being a Black woman in this medical system means knowing that you can do every-thing "right" and still be ignored. You can ask the right questions, advocate clearly, bring a partner, and still get dismissed. It's not in your head. It's not a fluke. It's what the data show over and over again.

Black women are more likely to have their pain undertreated. More likely to be misdiagnosed or not diagnosed at all. More likely to be blamed for their symptoms. More likely to die during or after childbirth, even when income and education are the same as white women.

This scenario is not about fear. It's about facts. And it's about power.

You have the right to demand better. You have the right to say, "I will not be ignored today."

It's exhausting that you even have to plan for this. That your survival depends on walking into an exam room with backup, receipts, and strategy. But this isn't about doing it perfectly. It's about protecting yourself in a system that too often refuses to do so.

This system wasn't built for your safety. But that doesn't mean you have to navigate it alone.

What to Expect and What to Look Out For

You are not being "too much" for advocating for yourself. You are not paranoid for bringing someone with you. You are not overreacting for noticing a pattern.

The medical system has long treated Black women as less credible, less sensitive to pain, and less deserving of comprehensive care. That's not a relic of the past. It still shows up today in how your pain is rated, how your fertility is treated, how your ques-tions are answered, how fast you're discharged from the emergency room, and whether your provider listens to your needs.

You have every right to protect yourself, to walk in prepared, and to expect more.

Here's what that might look like:

- Bringing a support person to appointments, not just for moral support—but as a witness and as an advocate
- Writing down your questions ahead of time and keeping a copy in your phone
- Asking your provider to document specific symptoms in your chart and reading the notes afterward

- Asking, "Can you explain your thought process for this diagnosis or recommendation?"
- Following up in writing if something felt wrong or dismissive

You can also ask directly about provider experience:

- "What has your experience been like caring for Black women in your practice?"
- "Do you track patient outcomes by race or identity?"
- "What steps do you take to address bias in care?"

Support Person Planning

Having someone in the room with you can shift the dynamic. Whether it's a partner, friend, parent, or doula, here are a few ways they can support you:

- Take notes during the visit.
- Interrupt if you're being rushed or interrupted.
- Say, "Can we pause and come back to that?"
- Ask clarifying questions.
- Be a second set of ears when decisions are being made.
- Offer validation afterward if things felt off.

You should brief your support person ahead of time:

"I want you to step in if I'm getting brushed off."
"Can you write down anything I need to follow up on?"
"If I freeze, can you say something on my behalf?"

This isn't about being dramatic. It's about recognizing the risk and the harm and staying safe.

What to Say

Use these as is or adjust them in your own voice:

"I need to make sure my symptoms are fully documented."
"I want to understand your reasoning. Can you walk me through it?"
"I've had care dismissed in the past. I need to be taken seriously today."
"I'm going to bring someone with me to help track what's said."
"This doesn't feel right. I'd like to pause and reconsider."
"I'd like a copy of my visit notes before I leave."

Black Maternal Mortality and What to Watch For in Emergencies

Black women in the United States are still three to four times more likely to die from pregnancy-related complications than white women—even when controlling for income, education, and insurance. It's not a personal failure. It's a systemic failure.

You can be healthy, informed, and prepared and still be ignored. You can flag concerning symptoms and still be told it's normal. This is why advocating for yourself isn't optional. It's protective. It's necessary. And it's not too much. That doesn't mean you should have to do this alone.

If you're pregnant or postpartum:

- Track symptoms early and document everything, even if it feels minor.
- Know the warning signs of preeclampsia, infection, and postpartum complications.
- Ask providers to explain their decisions, and to write them down in your chart.
- Bring a support person who's ready to advocate *with* you, not just *for* you.

Ask your provider directly:

- "What steps do you take to reduce racial disparities in maternal outcomes?"
- "How do you ensure Black patients receive timely and appropriate treatment?"

If the answers are defensive or dismissive that tells you something important.

You have every right to switch providers, even late in pregnancy, if something doesn't feel right. You can bring a doula, advocate, or support person into the room. You can request a second opinion. You can push back on care that feels rushed, dismissive, or unsafe. Your safety, comfort, and dignity are not negotiable, and you don't need to wait for a crisis to speak up.

If you're already in a crisis—if you're bleeding, in severe pain, or heading to the emergency room (ER)—your strategy might need to shift...

When Crisis Hits: Seeking Care In the ER

The emergency room (ER) is where systemic bias can turn dangerous. Black patients are more likely to be under-triaged, wait longer for pain treatment, and be discharged with serious symptoms unrecognized or untreated. Even in an emergency, you may still have to fight to be heard. That is not fair. But it is real.

When the stakes are this high, preparation and persistence are not optional. They are protective.

If you're going to the ER:

- Bring someone with you, if at all possible. Their presence alone can help shift the power dynamic and provide another set of eyes, ears, and voices in the room.
- Use clear, specific language. Do not minimize. Say exactly what is happening.
  - "I'm in severe pain—9 out of 10."
  - "I'm worried about preeclampsia."
  - "I'm experiencing heavy bleeding with clots."
  - "These symptoms are not normal for me."
- Ask directly for what you need and for what must be documented:
  - "Can you document that in my chart?"
  - "I don't feel safe being discharged."
  - "I'd like to speak with the attending physician."
  - "If I'm being discharged, I want the reason clearly documented."
- Escalation is not aggression. It is a safety tool. If your concerns are being minimized, escalate early and clearly. Ask to speak with the attending physician or the charge nurse. Say "I need a reassessment. My symptoms are worsening." Ask "What diagnoses are you actively ruling out right now?" Say "Can you repeat back what you understand my symptoms to be?"
- Advocate for your vital signs. Vitals are often dismissed or normalized incorrectly, and trends matter more than a single number.
  - "My blood pressure is not normal for me."
  - "Has my blood pressure been trending up or down?"
  - "Can you recheck my vitals before discharge?"
- Before leaving, make sure you have clear answers on the next steps.
  - "What symptoms mean I should return immediately?"
  - "What diagnoses were considered and ruled out?"
  - "What follow-up is required, and how soon?"
  - "Who do I contact if this worsens tonight?"

If your symptoms continue, worsen, or change, return immediately or go to a different hospital. Bring your discharge paperwork with you and say, "I was discharged, but my symptoms persisted or escalated." Returning is not failure. It is survival.

You are allowed to be firm. You are allowed to interrupt. You are allowed to repeat yourself. You are allowed to take up space. You do not have to stay calm to be taken seriously.

Your silence should not be the price of receiving care. Your advocacy should not be mistaken for aggression. Your life should not depend on how politely you ask to be saved.

Say what you need to say. Repeat it if necessary. The ER does not get a pass because the stakes are high. That is exactly when your voice matters most.

Pre-Visit Planning

Use this page to ground yourself before a visit, especially if you're walking in with history or hesitation.

What is this visit for?

- ☐ Annual exam
- ☐ New symptoms or pain
- ☐ Fertility or family planning
- ☐ Birth control consult
- ☐ Pregnancy care
- ☐ Something else: _____

What is my biggest concern going into this visit?

_____

What do I want to feel by the time I leave?

- ☐ Heard
- ☐ Respected
- ☐ Believed
- ☐ Supported
- ☐ Something else: _____

Who's going with me (if anyone)?

_____

Is there anything I want to write down or bring with me?

_____

_____

What's worth sharing: Pertinent history

_____

_____

You don't need to justify your experience to deserve good care, but sometimes offering context can shift the dynamic and help you feel more in control. You can say it, write it, or bring a printed page to hand over.

You can also list symptoms, history, and questions in advance. That helps keep you anchored even when things get emotional or feel rushed.

For Support People

They're walking into a system with a well-documented history of dismissing Black patients' pain and concerns. Your presence matters—not because they're not credible on their own, but because *the system often refuses to listen.*

In routine visits:

- **Acknowledge the burden.** It's not fair they have to prep this much to be taken seriously. Help them get ready without implying it's their job to fix racism.
- **Validate what they experience.** If something feels off, name it. Say, "You're not overreacting. That wasn't okay."
- **Support their boundaries.** Trust their instincts about providers, even if nothing dramatic happens. Discomfort is enough.
- If you're in the room:
  - Take notes.
  - Amplify their voice if they're being interrupted or ignored.
  - Say, "She already mentioned that." "Can you clarify that again for both of us?"
  - Make it clear their presence, safety, and dignity are nonnegotiable.

(continued)

(continued)

In emergency care:

- **Stay calm *and* clear-eyed.** You might need to raise the alarm if care is delayed or symptoms are downplayed.
- **Use specific language providers understand.** Say:
  - "She's in 9 out of 10 pain."
  - "We're concerned about preeclampsia."
  - "This bleeding is not normal for her."
- Push for next steps:
  - "Can you document that?"
  - "Who is the attending physician?"
  - "We're not comfortable leaving without clear answers."
- **Don't be afraid to interrupt.** That's not being rude—it's being protective.
- **Most important: mirror their urgency.** Show them you're taking it just as seriously as they are. Because you should be.

They're not overreacting. They're protecting themselves. In too many cases, Black patients aren't taken seriously until it's too late. Your presence helps make sure they're heard.

Scenario 5

Navigating Gynecological Care with a History of Trauma

Tools to reclaim control, set boundaries, and access care without abandoning yourself

This is complex and we don't talk about it enough. But you're not alone in it. So many people carry histories that shape how their bodies respond to reproductive healthcare. And the system has a long way to go to truly see you, to make space for your safety, and to earn your trust back.

Because here's the truth most providers don't say out loud: trauma doesn't disappear at the clinic door. It comes with you. It sits in the waiting room. It stiffens your shoulders during intake. It follows you into the room, into the stirrups, and through every minute someone is asking you to relax while your nervous system is screaming the opposite.

No one prepares you for what it's like to sit on an exam table and feel your body remember something that you've spent years trying to forget. Maybe it was a single experience. Maybe it was a pattern. Maybe you don't have all the words, but you know what it felt like—something taken from you, something pushed past your no, something that made your body feel like it didn't belong to you anymore. And then, somewhere down the line, it's all brought up again when someone says, "Time for your pelvic exam."

You are not broken for feeling that way. You are not overreacting. And you don't have to white-knuckle your way through care just to get what you need.

If You've Been Avoiding Care—You're Not Alone

If you've skipped appointments, delayed care, or avoided providers altogether because of what you've been through. You're not failing. You're surviving. Avoidance is a normal response to past trauma. Sometimes the safest thing your nervous system can do is say, "Not yet." That doesn't make you broken.

What Care Can Actually Look Like

You are allowed to tell your provider, "I have a history of trauma and would like to go slowly."

You are allowed to ask them to explain everything before they do it.

You are allowed to say no.

You are allowed to stop at any time, even mid-exam, even mid-sentence.

You are allowed to cry.

You are allowed to bring someone with you.

You are allowed to do what you need to feel safe.

You are allowed to meet a new provider the first time without doing a physical exam to ensure you feel comfortable.

You are allowed to ask for a single-dose anti-anxiety medication if you think you would benefit from that.

You don't owe your story, your details, or your history.

You Set the Tone

You know more than anyone how your body responds and what your triggers are.

If you know your anxiety spikes in the waiting room, call ahead and ask if there's a way to wait in your car until the room is ready.

If the exam room is triggering, ask to stay dressed until the provider arrives, or bring a support person with you. You can also ask to have a medical assistant as a chaperone in the room during the exam if that feels more comfortable for you.

You are not being "too much."

And if the provider doesn't respond well, if they roll their eyes, brush off your concerns, rush the exam, or skip consent, you have every right to stop the appointment.

You can say:

- "Actually, I think I need to pause and reschedule."
- "This isn't feeling right for me, and I'm not going to continue."
- "I'd like to get dressed and leave now."

What's Worth Sharing: Pertinent History

Sharing your history can be incredibly difficult. You don't have to say anything you're not ready to. You are in control here. But offering even a little context can help your provider support you with more care, more gentleness, and fewer assumptions.

Here are some pieces of history you might choose to share, only if and when you feel safe:

- A history of sexual assault or abuse
- Prior pelvic exams or procedures that were physically or emotionally distressing
- Anxiety, panic attacks, or dissociation during past medical visits
- Fear of pain or re-traumatization during exams
- Discomfort with stirrups, speculums, or specific positioning
- Difficulty with male providers or certain settings (e.g., bright lights, closed doors)
- Need for detailed explanations and slower pacing
- Past experiences of not being believed or having your no ignored
- Any triggers you're aware of (e.g., certain language, touch without warning)
- Support needs like bringing someone with you or staying dressed longer

How to Say It (If You Want To)

You get to decide what you share, when you share it, and how. That might mean telling your provider verbally, writing it down, or saying nothing at all. These are all valid ways to communicate and things that you can say:

- "I've had some difficult experiences in the past, and I need this visit to be as gentle and communicative as possible."
- "Please talk me through every step before you do anything—and check in before you move forward."

- "I don't want to do anything today that feels rushed or automatic. If I pause or tense up, please check in instead of pushing through."
- "I'd like to just talk today and come back for an exam if I feel ready."

Even a note passed at check-in or to the provider that says, "I have a trauma history and need a slower visit" is enough. You do not need to explain further if you don't want to.

Grounding and Coping Strategies

It's also okay to prepare yourself ahead of time with grounding tools.

Wear clothing that makes you feel safe.

Bring headphones with calming music or a podcast.

Breathe into your belly and let yourself come back to the room as often as you need.

Ask the provider if you can have your feet flat on the table instead of in stirrups if that feels better.

And if you're not ready? That's okay, too.

Sometimes just booking the appointment is the win.

Sometimes sitting in the parking lot is the win.

Sometimes telling your provider, "I'm not ready to do anything today. I just want to talk," is the most radical act of self-care you can offer your body.

If You Dissociate or Freeze During Care

Sometimes your body's way of staying safe is to check out. That might mean going still, going quiet, or feeling completely disconnected. It's not weakness—it's protection. And it's common for trauma survivors.

If you feel it happening, you can try the following:

- Focusing on your feet or the texture of the table beneath you
- Naming five things you see in the room
- Tapping a finger on the exam table or on your leg and bring your attention to that
- Asking your support person to talk you through what's happening or hold your hand

If you feel that you've already frozen or dissociated:

- Take the time you need to come back to yourself.
- Ask to sit up, get dressed, or move to a chair.
- You don't have to explain—"I need to stop" is enough.

The Myth of the "Good Patient"

There's a myth in medicine that the best patient is the compliant one.

But compliance is not the same as consent.

You are not difficult for having boundaries.

You are not inconvenient for needing care to come with compassion.

Your trauma is not a barrier to care. It's a reason to demand better.

You deserve a provider who knows how to hold space.

One who listens. One who doesn't flinch at your hesitation.

One who says, "We can go at your pace," and means it.

And if you haven't found that provider yet, keep looking.

They're out there. And you are worth the search.

When It's Bigger Than the Exam Room

This workbook is here to help you get through medical visits without abandoning yourself, but for many people, trauma doesn't just show up during a pelvic exam. It shows up everywhere the body remembers. It can live in your breath, your sleep, your relationships, your self-image. It can show up in the moments that seem the most ordinary: a partner's hand on your back, a routine check-in at your doctor's office, even the thought of pregnancy or birth.

Trauma can shape how safe you feel in your own body. For some, it means constantly scanning for threat, even when nothing's wrong. For others, it means feeling disconnected from sensation altogether, like you're watching yourself from a distance. The truth is, trauma isn't just a memory. It's a body experience. And it's deeply unfair that survivors are often expected to navigate health, intimacy, and motherhood inside systems that rarely understand that.

Maybe you're trying to figure out if you want kids and your body's history makes that question feel impossible to answer. Maybe you're partnered but afraid to be touched, because your body still associates closeness with danger. Maybe you're trying to reclaim pleasure after harm, or simply move through the world without flinching when someone reaches out to comfort you. Maybe you're exhausted from pretending you're fine. This isn't just about tolerating a medical visit. This is about your life and how you live it.

There isn't nearly enough conversation about how trauma weaves itself through care, sexuality, fertility, and parenting. Survivors are often told to "just relax" or "move on," but healing doesn't work that way. It's layered, nonlinear, and sometimes messy. And you deserve providers who understand that complexity. People who don't rush you, who ask permission before they touch you, and who know that consent isn't a one-time checkbox.

If you're not seeing a therapist but you trust your provider, they might be a good place to start. You can say something like, "I think I need support outside of this room. Can you recommend someone?" A trauma-informed clinician should take that seriously and offer referrals to therapists, survivor-centered organizations, or body-based healing spaces that help you reconnect with yourself on your own terms.

Support can look different for everyone. For some, that means therapy, especially with clinicians trained in trauma modalities like eye movement desensitization and reprocessing, somatic experiencing, or internal family systems. For others, it's about reconnecting with the body through movement: yoga, dance, breathwork, or grounding practices that rebuild a sense of safety inside your skin. Some people find comfort in survivor circles or group programs, where you can share your story and hear others say "me, too" in a space that believes you. And for others, healing begins with telling your story. Writing, creating, speaking, or finding small ways to give language to what happened so it doesn't keep living unspoken in your body.

Whatever form it takes, you get to choose what healing looks like for you. There's no right timeline, no done point, no checklist. Needing more support isn't a flaw, it's a sign that you're paying attention to what you actually need. You don't have to keep fighting through appointments, or intimacy, or life. You deserve care that extends beyond the table—care that helps you rebuild safety, rediscover connection, and remember that your body is still yours. Whole, worthy, and capable of healing.

Pre-Visit Planning

Use this space to prepare ahead of time so you don't have to explain everything in the moment.

What are you going in for?

☐ Annual exam
☐ Birth control consult
☐ Pain or symptoms
☐ Just to talk and get established
☐ Something else: _____

What feels hardest about this visit?

☐ Being touched
☐ Being undressed
☐ Being alone in the room
☐ Not feeling in control
☐ Something else: _____

What might help you feel safer?

☐ Bring a support person
☐ Stay dressed until provider enters
☐ Listen to music or use grounding tools
☐ Ask to skip the physical exam
☐ Something else: _____

What part of my history do I want to share:

_____

_____

How do I feel comfortable sharing this history?

_____

_____

For Support People

They're showing incredible courage by seeking care in settings that might trigger memories of powerlessness or violation. They need someone who understands that their body's responses aren't overreactions, they're protective mechanisms.

Honoring their courage. Validate that medical settings can feel scary after trauma. Celebrate every healthcare interaction they navigate, regardless of outcome.

Respecting their pace. Don't push them to "be okay" with something that felt wrong. Healing isn't linear, and their boundaries are always valid.

Supporting recovery. Help them process difficult appointments without pressure to forgive or forget. Their feelings about medical experiences are always legitimate.

If you're joining for the visit. Ask what they need and want from you. Be ready to provide support. Watch for signs they're distancing themselves from their body or shutting down. Be ready to help them stay present. Be ready to advocate for breaks or stopping the appointment if needed.

Scenario 6

Mental Health Deserves a Plan

Whether it's pregnancy-related, cycle-related, or always there in the background, your mental health matters—and deserves real care

Mental health isn't a side note. It's not an afterthought to your physical symptoms or something you only address when it starts interfering with your daily life. It's a core part of your health. Just as real, measurable, and deserving of care as your blood pressure, hormones, or Pap smear.

For many people, mental health challenges do not exist in isolation. They are woven through every stage of reproductive life, often shaped by events no one plans for and few people talk about. Hormones fluctuate. Identities shift. Responsibilities grow. And the world keeps moving faster than our capacity to rest or recover.

For some, symptoms intensify during pregnancy or postpartum. For others, they arrive like clockwork before a period or linger as a low, constant hum that never fully quiets. And for many, they are triggered or compounded by the unexpected: infertility and fertility treatments, pregnancy loss, abortion, complications during birth, a child's medical diagnosis, or the long-term emotional weight of caregiving. These experiences can disrupt a sense of control, safety, and identity in ways that are both profound and invisible.

Mental health is also shaped by grief that does not always have language. The loss of a hoped-for pregnancy. The loss of bodily trust after medical trauma. The loss of ease after becoming responsible for another life. Even moments that are supposed to be joyful can carry fear, exhaustion, or isolation alongside love.

None of this happens in a vacuum. It unfolds within bodies already navigating hormonal cycles and within systems that often fail to offer adequate support. Recognizing this complexity matters, because mental health symptoms are not personal failures or isolated diagnoses. They are often rational responses to layered stress, uncertainty, loss, and change.

Maybe you've always been "the anxious one," but lately your thoughts feel heavier, more intrusive, or harder to shake. Maybe you've never labeled what you're feeling as depression, but you recognize the exhaustion, irritability, or loss of interest that keeps showing up. Maybe you've had a baby and can't stop worrying about something happening to them. Or perhaps you can't find joy where you expected it. Maybe you feel fine one day and underwater the next, wondering if you're "just hormonal" or if something deeper is going on.

Here's the truth: it doesn't matter whether it's tied to your cycle, your pregnancy, your parenting, or your past, what matters is that it's real. You don't have to minimize it, explain it away, or prove it's "bad enough" to deserve care. If it's interfering with how you want to live, it's enough. You're enough.

This scenario is here to help you figure out what kind of support might be helpful, how to bring it up, and how to make sure you don't get dismissed, minimized, or left to figure it out alone. Whether you're navigating hormonal mood shifts, anxiety that peaks in waiting rooms, or depressive episodes that steal your energy for weeks at a time, there are tools, and people, who can help you find your way back to yourself.

In this scenario, we'll talk about the following:

- **I: Premenstrual syndrome (PMS) versus premenstrual dysphoric disorder (PMDD).** Understanding the difference between common premenstrual mood changes and premenstrual dysphoric disorder, and what kind of help each deserves.

- **II: Perinatal mental health (pregnancy and postpartum).** What it looks like, why perinatal anxiety and depression is more common than most people think, and how to ask for help early.

- **III: Navigating general anxiety and depression without a primary care provider (PCP).** How to bring it up with your OB-GYN, urgent care, or another provider when you don't have a primary doctor managing your care.

- **IV: Getting referrals to psychiatry and other mental healthcare.** When therapy or medication might be the next step, and how to make sure you're connected to someone who actually listens.

- **V: Using screening tools like the PHQ-9 to check in with yourself.** Because tracking symptoms over time can help you see patterns, communicate clearly with your provider, and catch changes before they spiral.

Your mental health deserves a plan. One that fits your life, your body, and your circumstances. This isn't about perfection or pretending to be fine. It's about being honest with yourself, asking for what you need, and understanding that tending to your mind is a radical act of care for your body.

I: PMS Versus PMDD

Many people experience some emotional or physical changes before their period—feeling a little more irritable, bloated, tired, or weepy in the days leading up to it. That's called *PMS*, and while it's uncomfortable, it usually doesn't stop you from functioning.

But when those symptoms go beyond mood swings or cramps. When they feel like they hijack your brain, your emotions, or your relationships, it might be something more serious: PMDD.

PMDD is a severe, cyclical form of depression that's directly linked to the hormonal changes in your menstrual cycle. The symptoms often show up about one to two weeks before your period and lift shortly after bleeding begins. They can include intense mood swings, rage or irritability, hopelessness, intrusive thoughts, or feeling out of control in your own body. Some people describe it as "falling off an emotional cliff" every month, only to climb back up again once their period starts.

Because the symptoms are tied to hormonal changes, PMDD often gets brushed off as "just bad PMS" or "being emotional." But here's the thing: it's not in your head and it's not something you can just "push through." PMDD is a real, diagnosable condition that affects an estimated 5–8% of menstruating people. And it deserves real treatment.

If you suspect what you're feeling might be PMDD, you can start by tracking your symptoms for at least two cycles. Note when they start, when they end, and how severe they feel. This helps your provider see the pattern and differentiate PMDD from depression or anxiety that might be ongoing.

Treatment for PMDD can include lifestyle adjustments, taking birth control continuously to suppress the fluctuations that trigger symptoms, or selective serotonin reuptake inhibitors (a type of antidepressant often used cyclically or daily). Some people also find relief through nutrition, exercise, mindfulness, and therapy, especially approaches that integrate mind-body awareness.

Bottom line: you shouldn't have to brace yourself for two weeks of every month. If your mood consistently crashes before your period and it's affecting your work, relationships, or self-esteem, it's worth bringing up. You deserve care that looks at your full cycle, not just your symptoms. The following table identifies the differences between PMS and PMDD.

PMS	PMDD
Mild to moderate symptoms	Severe mood swings, anger, depression
May feel bloated, tired, weepy	May have suicidal thoughts or major functional impairment
Usually doesn't interfere with daily life	Often interferes with work, relationships, sleep
Improves once period starts	Relieved when bleeding begins, but much more intense

If you think you may have PMDD, tracking your cycle and symptoms for at least two months is key. Bring that data to your provider and ask these questions:

- "Can we evaluate whether this could be PMDD?"
- "What treatment options exist: medications, therapy, lifestyle?"
- "Can I try cycle tracking or hormone-based treatment options?"

PMS or PMDD Reflection Questions

- What emotions do I tend to feel in the week or two before my period?

- Are these emotions mild and manageable? Or do they feel intense and disruptive?

- Do these symptoms affect my ability to work, sleep, or be in relationships?

- How quickly do they resolve once my period starts?

- Have I noticed patterns for at least two months in a row?

- Am I having thoughts that concern me about this time?

- Would I feel more in control if I tracked this over time?

- What would I like to ask a provider about managing this?

Two-Month Cycle Tracker: Spotting Patterns in PMS Versus PMDD

Use this tool to track emotional and physical symptoms over at least two full cycles. The goal is to identify patterns tied to your menstrual cycle, which is key in evaluating for PMDD.

Repeat this every few days or with a notable difference in mood for atleast two menstrual cycles. You may have to copy it on to your own paper for additional tracking. More data is better!

- **Cycle day.** Day 1 = first day of bleeding
- **Mood and physical symptoms.** Use icons or check boxes to track what you're experiencing
- **Daily Impact Scale**
  - 1 = No impact
  - 2 = Mild (you noticed, but got through the day)
  - 3 = Moderate (some disruption)
  - 4 = High (missed responsibilities, needed support)
  - 5 = Severe (couldn't function, crisis level)

Cycle Day	Mood Symptoms (mark all that apply)	Physical Symptoms (mark all that apply)	Daily Impact (1–5 scale)	Notes
	☐ Sadness ☐ Irritability ☐ Anxiety ☐ Tearful ☐ Rage ☐ Numbness ☐ other:_____	☐ Bloating ☐ Cramps ☐ Fatigue ☐ Headache ☐ Nausea ☐ Sleep issues ☐ other:_____		
	☐ Sadness ☐ Irritability ☐ Anxiety ☐ Tearful ☐ Rage ☐ Numbness ☐ other:_____	☐ Bloating ☐ Cramps ☐ Fatigue ☐ Headache ☐ Nausea ☐ Sleep issues ☐ other:_____		
	☐ Sadness ☐ Irritability ☐ Anxiety ☐ Tearful ☐ Rage ☐ Numbness ☐ other:_____	☐ Bloating ☐ Cramps ☐ Fatigue ☐ Headache ☐ Nausea ☐ Sleep issues ☐ other:_____		

Cycle Day	Mood Symptoms (mark all that apply)	Physical Symptoms (mark all that apply)	Daily Impact (1–5 scale)	Notes
	☐ Sadness ☐ Irritability ☐ Anxiety ☐ Tearful ☐ Rage ☐ Numbness ☐ other:_____	☐ Bloating ☐ Cramps ☐ Fatigue ☐ Headache ☐ Nausea ☐ Sleep issues ☐ other:_____		
	☐ Sadness ☐ Irritability ☐ Anxiety ☐ Tearful ☐ Rage ☐ Numbness ☐ other:_____	☐ Bloating ☐ Cramps ☐ Fatigue ☐ Headache ☐ Nausea ☐ Sleep issues ☐ other:_____		

Interpreting Your Patterns

- PMS tends to show up mildly one to seven days before your period, and symptoms fade with bleeding. It usually doesn't disrupt function.
- PMDD symptoms:
  - Start after ovulation (about day 14 before your period begins)
  - Peak in the 5–10 days before your period
  - Interfere with daily life (work, relationships, sleep)
  - Are gone or much better within a few days of bleeding starting

II: Perinatal Mental Health (Pregnancy and Postpartum)

Postpartum Support International's motto is simple but powerful: "You're not alone. You're not to blame. And with help, you will be well." I love this motto so much. Because no one tells you how overwhelming it can feel when your body, hormones, and identity are all shifting at once, and while people may tell you it will get better, it's hard to believe it when you're struggling.

Mental health during pregnancy and after birth is its own category, and it needs to be taken seriously. It's not just the "baby blues." The "baby blues" usually show up a few days after birth. It looks like crying easily, feeling overwhelmed, or having mood swings. And it tends to fade within about two weeks. But when those feelings last longer, intensify, or start affecting how you function, it's not just hormones balancing out. And it deserves care, not shame.

Up to one in five people experience perinatal mood and anxiety disorders, and the symptoms can look different for everyone. Some people feel sadness, guilt, or disconnection. Others feel constant anxiety, intrusive or scary thoughts, or flashes of rage that seem to come from nowhere. Some feel emotionally numb. Like they're going through the motions but not really *in* their life. Some can't sleep even when the baby's asleep; others want to sleep all the time. These symptoms can show up during pregnancy, after birth, or even months later.

Symptoms can include:

- Depression during or after pregnancy
- Anxiety or panic attacks
- Intrusive thoughts (often distressing, unwanted, or frightening)
- Irritability or rage
- Emotional numbness or disconnection
- Difficulty bonding with the baby or feeling like you're "faking it"
- Feeling unlike yourself or questioning your worth as a parent
- Suicidal ideation

None of this makes you a bad parent. It's incredibly common, yet laced in shame.

Unfortunately, our culture romanticizes motherhood while minimizing the realities of what it takes to get there and then doesn't support you once you've arrived to motherhood. There's pressure to be grateful, to bounce back, to love every minute. But healing, both physical and emotional, takes time. You deserve space to feel what's real without judgment.

If any of these symptoms sound familiar, **reach out sooner, not later**. Talk to your OB-GYN, midwife, primary care provider, or a therapist. Mention that you've been reading about perinatal mental health and you'd like to be screened. Even just saying, "I don't feel like myself and I need help," is a start.

There are also organizations built specifically for this:

- **Postpartum Support International (PSI)** offers free peer mentors, online support groups, and a help line you can call or text at 1-800-944-4773 (text "HELP" to 800-944-4773)
- **Therapists trained in perinatal mental health (PMH-C certified)** specialize in pregnancy, birth, and parenting transitions.

And if at any point you feel like you might hurt yourself or someone else, please don't wait—**call 911 or go to your nearest emergency room**. You can also call or text **988** to reach the **Suicide and Crisis Lifeline**, which is available 24/7 and can connect you to trained counselors right away.

You don't have to be in crisis alone. Help exists, and you deserve to receive it with the same urgency and compassion as any other medical emergency.

You are not a bad parent for feeling this way. You are not alone. And you deserve help.

Perinatal Mental Health Reflection Questions

- How have I been feeling emotionally during pregnancy or postpartum?

- Do I feel like myself? Or like a different version of me?

- Have I been more irritable, anxious, or angry than usual?

- Am I having thoughts that scare me, even if I wouldn't act on them?

- Am I struggling to bond with my baby or feel numb?

- Do I feel supported? Or alone and overwhelmed?

- What am I afraid to say out loud?

- What would it feel like to ask for help?

- Who in my life could support me in bringing this up?

III: Navigating Anxiety or Depression Without a PCP

Let's name the truth: having a PCP can make mental health support much easier. PCPs are often the ones who prescribe first-line medications for anxiety and depression, refer to therapy, manage follow-up care, and help monitor how treatment is working over time. But not everyone has a PCP. And not having one doesn't mean you're out of options.

If you're already seeing an OB-GYN or reproductive care provider, they can often help bridge the gap. Many OB-GYNs are comfortable prescribing antidepressants or anxiety medications, especially for people who are postpartum, going through hormonal shifts, or dealing with reproductive-related mental health issues. Even if their training isn't centered in mental healthcare, they might be your best entry point for support right now.

You can ask these questions:

- "Would you feel comfortable prescribing medication or helping me get started?"
- "Can you refer me to a therapist or mental health clinic?"
- "Is there someone in your office who can help me navigate mental health support while I look for a PCP?"
- "Can you help me get connected to a PCP who manages mental healthcare?"

Asking for a PCP referral is important, especially if you know you'll need longer-term support. It doesn't mean you're closing the door on OB-GYN support, but it opens the door to more consistent, comprehensive care. And ask early. Often PCPs can take several months to get in, and you don't want to be scrambling.

And if you're not sure whom you *should* be looking for next, the following section will walk you through it: how to know when you might need a therapist, a psychiatrist, or both. You don't have to figure this out alone, and you don't have to wait for it to get worse before asking for help.

IV: Getting Referrals to Psychiatry and Other Mental Healthcare

Sometimes, mental health support means more than talking to your OB-GYN or getting a prescription from your PCP. You might need a therapist to talk through things over time. You might need a psychiatrist to help with medication, diagnostic clarity, or complex symptoms. And sometimes? You might need both.

What's the Difference Between Therapy and Psychiatry?

- **Therapists** (including psychologists, social workers, and counselors) focus on talk therapy. They help you work through emotions, trauma, relationships, and patterns over time. Some specialize in things like pregnancy, trauma, or grief. They can't prescribe medication, but they're often the front line of mental healthcare.
- **Psychiatrists** (and some psychiatric nurse practitioners or physician associates) are medical providers who can prescribe medication and manage complex psychiatric conditions. They're especially helpful when symptoms are severe, persistent, or unclear, or when therapy alone hasn't been enough.

You don't need to pick one or the other right away. But if you're not currently seeing either, your OB-GYN or PCP can help you figure out what's needed based on what you're experiencing.

What You Can Say

If you're not sure what you need but you know you need *something*, it's okay to start the conversation anyway.

You can say the following:

- "I'm not currently seeing a therapist, but I'd like to."
- "Can you help me get connected to someone for talk therapy?"
- "Do you have referrals for mental health professionals who work with pregnancy, postpartum, or trauma?"
- "I think I need both medication and therapy. Can we build the right team together?"
- "Is there someone in your office who can help me find a good fit or sort through my insurance?"

Why It's Hard—and Why That's Not On You

Mental health access is a mess in many parts of the country. It can take weeks or months to find a therapist or psychiatrist who can do the following:

- Accept new patients
- Is covered by your insurance
- Is culturally competent or trauma-informed
- Is available outside of traditional 9–5 hours
- Is a good personality fit

That doesn't mean you're asking for too much. That means the system isn't designed for how common these needs actually are.

Planning Ahead—Even If the Wait Is Long

Getting on the list *now* is better than waiting until you're in crisis. Here's how to make progress:

- Ask for multiple names or practices in case one doesn't pan out
- Start the insurance search early. Call your insurance company or use their provider portal
- Consider virtual options
- Ask if your OB-GYN office has a mental health coordinator or social worker to help connect you
- Tell a trusted provider if you're overwhelmed by the search and ask for help navigating it

If you're trying to find therapy for the first time, you can say the following:

- "I don't know where to start. Can someone help me with this?"
- "Can I get a few referrals for therapists who specialize in _____?" (anxiety, post-partum, trauma, etc.)

Red Flags to Watch For

If a provider ignores or downplays your mental health concerns, that's not a reflection of your need, it's a sign they might not be the right person to guide you.

If you hear:

- "We don't really handle that here."
- "That's just stress, try getting more sleep."
- "You don't seem that bad."

You're allowed to say:

- "I'm asking for a referral because I don't want it to get worse."
- "Even if it doesn't seem urgent to you, it feels important to me."
- "Can we treat this like any other health issue and take the next step?"

Whether you're looking for someone to talk to, someone to prescribe, or someone who can help *figure it out with you*, you're allowed to ask for a team. You don't need a diagnosis to deserve care. You don't have to wait until you're falling apart to speak up.

Mental healthcare isn't a luxury. It's part of your whole health. And building the right support system is one of the strongest things you can do.

Baseline: How I'm Doing Right Now

How have I been feeling emotionally in the past month?

Do I notice getting worse around my period (if applicable)?

Have I been feeling this way for a while, or is this new?

Do I have a provider I feel comfortable talking to about this if needed?

☐ Yes   ☐ No   ☐ Not sure

V: Using Screening Tools Like the PHQ-9 to Check In with Yourself

The PHQ-9 (Patient Health Questionnaire-9) is a trusted, evidence-based screening tool used by healthcare providers to assess symptoms of depression. It's quick. It's simple. And it can be a powerful first step in recognizing when something is off.

This tool is not a diagnosis—but it can be a signal that your mental health deserves more attention.

When to Use It

You might want to take the PHQ-9 if the following is true:

- You've been feeling low, irritable, numb, or unlike yourself for more than a few days.
- You're not sure if what you're experiencing "counts" as depression.
- You're in a postpartum period or major life transition.
- You're preparing for a visit and want to bring something tangible to your provider.
- You're tracking symptoms over time to see if they're getting better or worse.

This isn't just a test for crisis. It's a check-in for your mental and emotional baseline.

If you'd like to complete the PHQ9, answer the following based on how often you've been bothered by each problem in the last two weeks.

Scoring:

- 0 = Not at all
- 1 = Several days
- 2 = More than half the days
- 3 = Nearly every day

Question	Scoring
1. Little interest or pleasure in doing things	
2. Feeling down, depressed, or hopeless	
3. Trouble falling or staying asleep, or sleeping too much	
4. Feeling tired or having little energy	
5. Poor appetite or overeating	
6. Feeling bad about yourself—or that you're a failure or have let yourself or your family down	
7. Trouble concentrating on things, such as reading or watching TV	
8. Moving or speaking so slowly that other people could have noticed—or the opposite: being so fidgety or restless that you were moving a lot more than usual	
9. Thoughts that you would be better off dead, or thoughts of hurting yourself in some way	

Your Total Score = _____

How to Interpret Your Score—Depression Severity

- **0–4 (minimal).** You may not need clinical intervention, but keep checking in with yourself. You're allowed to take your mental health seriously even at a "low" score.
- **5–9 (mild).** It's worth having a conversation with a provider or therapist. Early support can prevent things from getting worse.
- **10–14 (moderate).** Time to reach out. You may benefit from therapy, medication, or both—and it's absolutely okay to ask for help.
- **15–19 (moderately severe).** Please don't wait. This level of symptom severity deserves professional care and consistent follow-up.
- **20–27 (severe).** This is serious. Your well-being matters too much to push through this alone. Contact a provider immediately—or go to the nearest clinic or emergency room if you feel unsafe.

★★If you answered anything other than 0 on question 9 (thoughts of self-harm): This is a priority concern. Please don't try to carry it on your own.

→ **Call or text 988 (Suicide and Crisis Lifeline).**
→ Tell someone you trust.
→ Reach out to a provider today.

How Often Should You Retake It?

- Retake it every several weeks if you're monitoring symptoms over time.
- Use it before a visit to help advocate for the level of support you need.
- Bring it to a new provider if you're establishing mental healthcare and want a way to communicate how you've been feeling.

Mental health is dynamic. Just like your physical health, it changes, and it's okay to track it.

This tool isn't the whole picture. But it's a starting point. And sometimes, that's exactly what you need.

Pre-Visit Planning

Before your appointment, take a few minutes to center yourself. What's been weighing on you? What kind of support are you hoping for? Use this space to gather your thoughts, especially if talking about mental health feels vulnerable or overwhelming.

What I want to bring up during this visit:

How my mental health has been feeling lately:

What I'm hoping to get from this appointment *(check all that apply):*

- ☐ A space to talk about what I'm experiencing
- ☐ Guidance on whether therapy might help
- ☐ Information about medication options
- ☐ A referral to a therapist or psychiatrist
- ☐ Support for perinatal or cycle-related mental health
- ☐ A screening tool like the PHQ-9
- ☐ Help figuring out what kind of care I need

I feel nervous about bringing this up because:

_____

_____

It would help me if my provider:

- ☐ Gave me space to talk without judgment
- ☐ Took my symptoms seriously
- ☐ Helped me understand next steps
- ☐ Reassured me that I'm not alone

Final Mental Health Note: You Deserve Support

Mental health is part of your reproductive health and part of your whole health. Whether you're managing anxiety that's always been there, navigating depression after birth, or just starting to notice that your cycle seems to knock you off balance every month, your experience is valid. And it's worth paying attention to.

You don't have to have a diagnosis to deserve support. You don't have to wait until it gets worse. And you don't have to go through it alone.

You are not a burden for needing help.

You are not weak for feeling overwhelmed.

You are not broken.

You are human.

And you deserve care that sees the whole you.

For Support People

They may be struggling to advocate for themselves while dealing with depression, anxiety, or other mental health challenges. They need someone who takes their emotional well-being as seriously as any physical symptom and won't let it be dismissed as "just stress."

Normalizing mental healthcare. Help them recognize that mental health *is* healthcare. Their emotional well-being deserves the same care, attention, and follow-up as anything else in their medical chart.

Stigma smashing matters. Medication for mental health is not a failure. It's a tool. Just like insulin for diabetes or a cast for a fracture. If they're exploring

(continued)

(continued)

antidepressants or other prescriptions, talk about it like you would any other treatment. You can say things like, "That's a smart step" or "I'm proud of you for taking care of yourself." Your words matter more than you know.

Supporting the journey. Be patient with the ups and downs of mental health treatment. It's not always linear. Celebrate the good days, show up on the hard ones, and offer calm reassurance when they feel overwhelmed or discouraged. Stability is its own form of love.

Practical assistance. If they're struggling with brain fog, fatigue, or anxiety, offer help with logistics: writing down questions, managing medications, finding a therapist, or making appointments. Just remember: support doesn't mean control. Ask before stepping in.

If you're joining for the visit. Don't let providers separate mental and physical health, or brush off emotional symptoms as less important. Help validate their experience if they freeze, forget, or struggle to articulate what's going on. You can say, "We're hoping for support that takes both physical and mental health into account."

If they're having thoughts of self-harm. Take it seriously. Stay calm. Ask directly but gently, "Are you safe right now?" and "Do you have a plan to hurt yourself?"

If the answer is yes, or even *maybe*, **do not leave them alone.** Sit with them. Stay on the phone. Be a steady presence. Then take action: call or text **988 (Suicide and Crisis Lifeline)** or help them get to a safe place. You don't need to know the perfect words. You just need to stay.

If there are firearms or other lethal means at home, make a safety plan immediately. Remove access or store them securely. This step could save their life.

Safety is not an overreaction. It's not shameful. It's love in its most urgent form.

CYCLE SYMPTOMS, HORMONAL SHIFTS, INFECTIONS, AND PAIN CONCERNS

Scenario 7

Birth Control That Works For You

Whether you're starting, stopping, or switching—this is how to own the conversation

A Quick Note Before You Go In

Birth control is powerful. It gives you options, freedom, and control over your body and your future. But too often, the way it's offered doesn't feel like a choice, it feels like an assumption. Like the method was picked for you. Or like wanting something different makes you difficult.

You deserve better.

Whether you're starting birth control for the first time, switching methods, or coming off it entirely, you're allowed to make the choice that fits you. You're allowed to ask questions, take your time, and expect respect. This isn't about being "for" or "against" birth control. It's about making sure the method works for you—not the other way around.

And here's something that doesn't get said enough: *there's no such thing as being on birth control "too long."* The science doesn't support the idea that using hormonal contraception for years somehow "builds up" or harms fertility. What matters most is whether it still fits your body, your goals, and your life right now.

So how do you decide what's right for you?

Start by thinking about your goals:

- Do you need the highest level of pregnancy prevention?
- Are you okay with some risk?
- Do you want something hormonal or nonhormonal?
- Are you managing more than pregnancy prevention? Painful periods, mood swings, acne, or irregular bleeding?

Every method has different typical use efficacy (real-world results) and perfect use efficacy (best-case results). You'll find a comparison chart in this section to help you sort through those options. You'll also see the phrase *risk threshold for pregnancy* throughout. Because this isn't black-and-white. Some people want the most effective method possible. Others are fine with a little risk. Your comfort zone matters.

And if you need birth control that a partner or parent won't see or know about, consider a LARC (long-acting reversible contraceptive), like an intrauterine device (IUD) or implant. These are private, discreet, and do not require regular refills. But if you are on a parent's insurance, be aware that insurance billing can generate explanations of benefits (EOBs) that may be visible to the policyholder. For some people, this means exploring options outside of insurance or asking a clinic about confidentiality protections or cash pricing, depending on what feels safest and most accessible for you.

Birth Control Isn't Only About Preventing Pregnancy

Birth control is often prescribed for other reasons, including the following:

- Regulating heavy or painful periods
- Managing premenstrual syndrome (PMS) or premenstrual dysphoric disorder (PMDD)
- Improving hormonal acne
- Controlling bleeding with polycystic ovary syndrome (PCOS) or endometriosis
- Helping with perimenopause symptoms

What About What I See Online?

Let's name something that's been happening: birth control has been getting a lot of negative attention online. You may see claims that it causes infertility, disconnects you from your body, or permanently harms your health. Some people share real experiences of side effects that led them to stop using birth control, and those experiences deserve to be taken seriously. Not every method works for every body, and listening to people when something does not feel right matters.

What becomes a problem is when individual experiences are turned into blanket claims that birth control is inherently bad or dangerous. That kind of framing often relies on fear rather than evidence and leaves people without the full picture they need to make informed choices.

Birth control is not dangerous, shameful, or anti-feminist. It is a medical tool. For generations, it has helped people plan their families, pursue education, protect their health, and make decisions about their own lives. Reframing it as universally harmful or oppressive ignores how transformative it has been for millions of people who finally had agency over their futures.

You can support access to birth control and still decide it is not right for you.

You can trust your body and still use hormonal contraception.

You can question your options and still choose a method that helps you feel like yourself.

What you deserve is full, balanced information, not pressure or fear from any direction.

Birth Control Myths

Just because you see it online does not mean it is true.

Myth	What's Actually True
"Birth control makes you infertile."	Most methods are fully reversible.
"Hormones build up in your body."	They don't. Your body processes them continuously.
"If it doesn't work for you, something's wrong with you."	No. It might just not be the right fit. That's data, not failure.
"Natural = better."	Natural isn't always easier or more effective. It's a choice, not a moral high ground.

Choosing a Method: Quick Comparison of the Most Common Methods

Not every method is safe for every person, especially if you have migraines with aura, high blood pressure, blood clotting disorders, or smoke over age 35. If any of these apply, tell your provider so they can tailor your options.

Method	Efficacy Typical Use → Perfect Use	Pregnancy Risk	Ease of Use	Hormonal?	Used for More Than Pregnancy?	Typical Side Effects
Pill	~91% → 98%	Moderate unless perfect use	Daily pill—requires consistency	Yes	Yes—acne, cycles, mood	Nausea, breast tenderness, mood changes, break-through bleeding
Implant (Nexplanon)	Over 99%	Extremely low	One-time insertion, lasts three to five years	Yes	Yes—periods, cramps, acne	Irregular bleed-ing, mood changes, possible weight gain
IUD (hormonal)	Over 99%	Extremely low	Inserted once, lasts three to eight years	Yes	Yes—bleeding, cramps	Irregular or lighter bleeding, cramping after insertion
IUD (copper)	Over 99%	Extremely low	Inserted once, lasts 10+ years	No	No—Sometimes worsens bleeding/cramps	Heavier periods, more cramping, especially early on
Shot (Depo)	~94%	Low	Every three months	Yes	Yes—periods, pain	Irregular bleed-ing, delayed return to fertility, weight gain
Patch	~91% → 98%	Moderate	Weekly patch change	Yes	Yes	Skin irritation, nausea, breast tenderness
Ring (NuvaRing)	~91% → 98%	Moderate	Monthly ring placement	Yes	Yes	Vaginal discharge, spotting, breast tenderness

Method	Efficacy Typical Use → Perfect Use	Pregnancy Risk	Ease of Use	Hormonal?	Used for More Than Pregnancy?	Typical Side Effects
Condoms	~82% → 95%	Moderate to high	Use every time, user-dependent	No	Yes—sexually transmitted infection (STI) prevention	Latex allergy (if applicable), reduced sensation
Fertility Awareness— Including cycle tracking app	Average ~76% →95–99% with precision	High unless used precisely	Requires daily tracking, discipline	No	Yes—body awareness, cycle insight, symptom tracking	None, but requires daily effort and cycle literacy
Tubal ligation/ removal	Over 99%	Permanent solution	Surgical procedure, outpatient	No	No	Cramping, fatigue post-op, surgical risks; may reduce cancer risk if tubes are removed
Partner vasectomy	Over 99% (after clearance)	Permanent solution	Outpatient procedure for partner	No	No	Mild swelling, soreness; requires follow-up semen test to confirm effectiveness
Withdrawal/ pull-out method	~74% → 95%	High unless used precisely	Requires awareness and timing with every encounter	No	No	None physically, but high risk of error; requires partner trust and communication

How to use this table:

- If you *absolutely do not want to get pregnant,* aim for methods with > 99% efficacy and low user dependence (like IUDs or implants) or combine two methods such as birth control pills and condoms.
- If you're *okay with a little risk,* you might prefer a method you can stop easily, like the pill or patch.
- If you want additional *noncontraceptive benefits,* look for hormonal methods that support acne, mood, or heavy bleeding.
- If you're managing a *chronic condition* (like endometriosis, PCOS, or PMDD), some methods may be recommended long-term, and that's totally okay.
- If you're *in a rural area* or have trouble accessing clinics, consider methods that last longer or don't require monthly refills.

Pre-Visit Planning

This section walks you through questions to ask and things to think about as you navigate your birth control journey. How to go on, switch, or come off birth control with clarity and support. You'll find tools to help you weigh your options, prepare for your appointment, ask thoughtful questions in the room, and lean on scripts if you face pushback.

Track 1: Going On Birth Control

Your why:

Reasons I'm considering starting birth control:

What I hope birth control will help with (pregnancy prevention, cycle control, acne, pain, mood, etc.):

Any concerns or hesitations I want to talk through with my provider:

Questions to ask:

- What are the side effects or benefits I should consider?
- How do different methods affect mood, weight, libido, or bleeding?
- Are there any red flags I should watch for in the first few weeks/months of use?
- How important is privacy or discretion in my current situation? (Do I need a method that a partner, parent, or insurance holder won't see?)
- Which methods are most reversible if I change my mind later?

- What should I know about long-term use or future fertility?
- What's available if I don't want hormones?
- Will this method also help manage anything else—like my period, acne, or mood?
- Is this covered by insurance or available at low/no cost? (Are there telehealth or mail-order options if in-person access is hard?)

Methods I'm interested in discussing:

☐ Pill

☐ Patch

☐ Ring

☐ IUD (hormonal)

☐ IUD (nonhormonal)

☐ Implant

☐ Shot

☐ Diaphragm or cervical cap

☐ Condoms or internal barrier methods

☐ Fertility awareness/cycle tracking

☐ Emergency contraception

☐ Sterilization

☐ Other: _____

My risk threshold for pregnancy:

☐ I absolutely do not want to get pregnant—highest efficacy is a priority.

☐ I'm okay with low risk.

☐ I'm okay with moderate risk.

☐ I'm open to pregnancy in the near future.

Rural considerations:
Long-acting methods (IUD, implant) may be worth prioritizing if your provider is hours away. Also ask about emergency contraception availability at pharmacies, mail-order options for pills, and what to do if you need urgent removal of a device.

Track 2: Switching Birth Control

Your why:

Reasons I'm considering switching my current method:

_____

Side effects I'm currently experiencing:

_____

Challenges with my current method (routine, access, etc.):

_____

Any methods I know I do *not* want:

_____

What I want my provider to understand about me and my goals:

_____

Am I switching because of provider suggestions, peer pressure, social media influence, or simply because I want something different?

_____

My risk threshold for pregnancy:

☐ I absolutely do not want to get pregnant—highest efficacy is a priority.
☐ I'm okay with low risk.
☐ I'm okay with moderate risk.
☐ I'm open to pregnancy in the near future.

Questions to ask:

- Are there methods with fewer side effects for me?
- Which options are easiest to stop or switch if needed?
- Can I change methods without a gap in protection?
- What's the adjustment period like with this new method?
- How quickly do side effects go away after switching?

Track 3: Coming Off Birth Control

Your why:

Reasons I want to come off birth control:

_____

Concerns I want to talk through with my provider:

_____

My risk threshold for pregnancy:

☐ I absolutely do not want to get pregnant. Highest efficacy is a priority.

☐ I'm okay with low risk.

☐ I'm okay with moderate risk.

☐ I'm open to pregnancy in the near future.

Questions to ask:

- What should I expect when stopping this method?
- How long might it take for my cycle to regulate?
- Are there any symptoms I should watch for?
- Can we make a plan for follow-up if anything feels off?

If You Get Pushback

You deserve to have your choices respected, no matter where you are in your birth control journey. If a provider resists your request, you can say the following:

- "I've made this decision."
- "Please document my request, even if you disagree."
- "If I change my mind, I'll come back."

You are the ultimate decision-maker in your reproductive care. Your provider's role is to offer guidance, not permission.

For Support People

They're making decisions about their body and future while navigating a system that often assumes what's best for them, rather than listening to their actual needs and preferences. They need someone who respects their autonomy completely and won't impose their own opinions about what method is "best."

Respecting their choices. Support their birth control decisions without judgment, even if you'd choose differently. Their body, their life, their choice. Always.

Method transitions. Be patient during adjustment periods. New methods can affect mood, energy, or physical comfort in ways that affect your relationship. Show up with compassion, not commentary.

Access support. Help with practical stuff—insurance hassles, pharmacy issues, or transportation to appointments—especially if they're switching methods or need timely refills.

If you're joining for the visit. Let them lead the conversation. Your role is to support, not to speak for them. Step back unless they ask you to step in.

For Sexual Partners

If you're sexually active with someone using birth control, you're part of the picture, even if it's not your body.

Contraception is not their responsibility alone. Ask how you can help, share the mental load, and listen to their boundaries. This includes learning about their cycle and being willing to track it too, rather than leaving all fertility awareness and planning on them. Never pressure someone to change methods based on your preferences.

Don't assume their method means "no risk." If pregnancy is a shared concern, talk about what you both need to feel safe and supported. This includes being open to using condoms, STI testing, and what your plan would be if a method fails.

Be honest and present. Trust and intimacy are built through shared decisions, not assumptions.

Scenario 8

Break-Through Bleeding That Doesn't Make Sense

Irregular bleeding, spotting after sex, periods that won't stop—and no clear answers

You're not pregnant. But something feels off.

You're bleeding between cycles. Spotting after sex. Or your period's lasting way longer than it used to. Maybe you've always been regular but now you're suddenly not. And no one's given you a real answer.

Breakthrough bleeding, whether it's mid-cycle spotting, post-sex bleeding, or periods that just won't stop, is one of the most common reasons people seek OB-GYN care. But it's also one of the easiest to dismiss, especially if you're told it's "just hormones," "stress," or "nothing to worry about." Sometimes that's true, but sometimes, it's not.

Abnormal bleeding can be caused by something simple, like a change in birth control or a small cervical polyp. But it can also be the body's way of waving a red flag. Persistent or unexplained bleeding can point to infections, fibroids, thyroid issues, endometrial changes, or precancerous or cancerous cells on the cervix or uterus. It doesn't mean you have something serious, but it does mean it's worth checking. The goal isn't panic. It's clarity.

If you notice bleeding that's new for you, track it. Write down when it happens, how long it lasts, what it looks like, and whether it follows sex, exercise, or stress. Note any new medications, supplements, or birth control changes too. Patterns tell stories. And when you can describe yours clearly, you make it harder for anyone to brush off your concern.

This scenario is for anyone who's bleeding when they shouldn't. You don't have to walk in knowing what's wrong. You just have to be able to say, "This isn't normal for me and I want to understand why it's happening." Because when something changes in your body, it's okay to ask questions.

What Might Be Going On?

Bleeding that's prolonged, shows up between periods, or starts after sex can be caused by a range of things. Some are hormonal. Some structural. Some related to infection, inflammation, or medications. Here are a few examples that providers often evaluate for:

- **Fibroids.** These are noncancerous growths in the uterus that can cause heavy or prolonged bleeding, including during times you wouldn't expect it.
- **Thyroid issues.** Both hypothyroidism and hyperthyroidism can affect bleeding and timing, sometimes leading to breakthrough or prolonged flow.
- **Birth control changes.** New hormonal methods, or missing pills—can cause unexpected spotting or continuous bleeding.
- **Sexually transmitted infections (STIs) or other infections.** Bleeding after sex or between periods can be a sign of inflammation or infection (like chlamydia, gonorrhea, or bacterial vaginosis). These are common and treatable.
- **Endometrial polyps or cervical irritation.** These are structural causes that may lead to bleeding with sex or spotting between periods.
- **Other causes.** These include medications, blood clotting conditions, recent surgeries, or even rough sex.
- **Or something scary.** In rarer cases, abnormal bleeding can signal precancerous or cancerous changes of the cervix, uterus, or endometrium. That's why evaluation matters—not to assume the worst, but to rule it out early if it's there.

If It Bothers You, Bring It Up

When your bleeding feels unpredictable or out of place, it can throw everything off. Your comfort, your confidence, your plans.

Sometimes it's nothing, but sometimes it means your body is signaling something, and that deserves attention. It is worth it to keep in mind that a one-time instance does not necessarily need a full workup. Keep your eyes on it. And if it's happening more than one cycle in a row, or it's starting to interfere with your life, tracking it helps you advocate clearly and push for answers.

When It Might Be Urgent

Breakthrough or prolonged bleeding can be disruptive, but sometimes, it's more than that.

Seek care more urgently if you experience any of the following:

- Bleeding so heavy you soak through a pad or tampon in under an hour for more than two hours
- Dizziness, extreme fatigue, or signs of anemia (like shortness of breath or a racing heart)
- Severe pelvic pain with bleeding
- Foul-smelling discharge, fever, or chills
- Bleeding after a known or suspected pregnancy
- Bleeding after menopause (even light spotting)

Pre-Visit Planning

Symptom Tracker: Help You and Your Provider See the Full Picture

Use this chart to track what you've been noticing. It doesn't have to be perfect, just consistent enough to show patterns. The goal isn't precision; it's perspective. Tracking helps you notice changes over time and gives your provider a clearer picture of what's happening and how it's affecting you. The more detail you can share, the easier it is to connect the dots together.

Symptom	Experiencing it? (✓)	How Often? (e.g., every cycle, randomly)	Impact on Life (1 = minimal, 10 = severe)	Notes
Spotting between periods				
Bleeding after sex				
Periods lasting more than seven days				

(continued)

Symptom	Experiencing it? (✓)	How Often? (e.g., every cycle, randomly)	Impact on Life (1 = minimal, 10 = severe)	Notes
Flow that seems nonstop or continuous				
Clots larger than a quarter				
Heavy flow (bleeding through pads/tampons in under an hour)				
Clots larger than a quarter				
Pelvic pressure or fullness				
Unexpected vaginal discharge or odor				
Bloating				
Bleeding after medication change/ viral illness				

What to Ask in the Exam Room

You may not get to every question. Star the ones that matter most to you. You're allowed to take notes or ask for time to think before deciding on a next step.

Initial questions:

- What could be causing this type of bleeding in my case?
- Is this common with my birth control or hormonal method?
- Should we check for fibroids, polyps, or signs of infection?

Testing and evaluation:

- Do I need bloodwork, STI testing, or a Pap today?
- Will a pelvic ultrasound help rule things out?
- Can you check for cervical changes or irritation?
- Could this be related to a thyroid issue?

If I'm on birth control or hormones:

- Is my current method contributing to the bleeding?
- Are there other options that might help stabilize it?
- If I switch methods, how long should I give it to regulate?

Next steps:

- If everything comes back normal, what's the plan?
- Is it okay to wait, or should we follow up after a set time?
- How long is too long for this kind of bleeding?
- Are there treatments that can help even if we don't find a clear cause?

What's Worth Sharing: Pertinent History

Bring this context with you, it helps your provider connect the dots.

Cycle history:

When was your last "normal" period?

_____

_____

How long have the irregularities been happening?

_____

_____

Do you bleed in between periods? After sex?

_____

_____

How many days are you bleeding? How heavy is it?

_____

_____

Impact on daily life:

☐ Missed work/school

☐ Worn pads + tampons + backup protection

☐ Avoided sex or intimacy

☐ Changed clothing routines or social plans

☐ Anxiety or stress around unpredictability

☐ Other

Medical history clues:

- Do you have a family history of fibroids, polycystic ovary syndrome, or thyroid disease?

_____

_____

- Are you currently on birth control or hormone therapy?

_____

_____

- Have you had any recent medication changes? Illnesses? Vaccinations? Higher stress levels?

_____

_____

- Any new partners since your last STI test?

_____

_____

Other clues to mention:

- Any new or worsening pelvic pressure or pain?

  _____

  _____

- Trouble with weight changes, facial/body hair growth, or acne?

  _____

  _____

- Any fatigue, temperature changes, or hair loss (possible thyroid)?

  _____

  _____

Use this space to clarify *why* you're coming in now. What's changed? What are you worried about?

_____

_____

_____

For Support People

They're dealing with bleeding that's unpredictable, disruptive, and often dismissed by a medical system that still treats irregular periods as "just one of those things." They need someone who takes their concerns seriously and stands with them—not someone who minimizes what they're going through.

Validate the disruption. Unpredictable bleeding can affect everything—from work and intimacy to mental health and daily routines. Acknowledge how exhausting that is. Help them adapt without making them feel like a burden.

Support them where they are. If this is a new issue, be patient while they gather information and figure out if it's a pattern. But if it's been going on for a while, help them look for answers—not just ways to cope. Support them in asking bigger questions, seeking second opinions, or pushing for testing if needed.

Hold space for the emotional weight. They may feel frustrated, embarrassed, or out of control—especially if their body isn't doing what it used to. Remind them this isn't their fault. They're allowed to want clarity. They're allowed to ask for more.

Offer practical backup. Keep extra supplies handy. Be flexible with plans. Help reduce the day-to-day friction that comes with never knowing what their body's going to do next.

If you're joining the visit. Let them lead. Be their second set of ears. And if they're being brushed off, help them push for real answers—not just "come back in a few months."

Scenario 9

Irregular Periods, PCOS, and Getting Real Answers

When your cycle is chaos, your symptoms are real, and "just go on the pill" isn't the answer you need

Your period doesn't have to be perfect, but it shouldn't be a mystery either. When it's been months since your last one, or when it shows up every few weeks, or when it's so heavy you're planning your life around it, that's not something to just "manage" with birth control and hope for the best.

But here's what often happens: you mention irregular periods, and you get handed a prescription for the pill. No questions about *why* your cycles are irregular. No discussion of what else might be going on. Just a quick fix that masks the problem instead of addressing it.

That's not healthcare. That's a bandage.

The truth is, irregular periods can be a sign of several different things: polycystic ovary syndrome (PCOS), thyroid issues, insulin resistance, stress, major weight changes, or other hormonal imbalances. And yes, birth control can help regulate your cycle and protect your uterine lining—but it doesn't always get to the root cause.

Still, let's be clear: there's no shame or shade in using birth control. For some people, it's exactly the right tool to manage symptoms, protect against pregnancy, or simply make life more predictable. The goal isn't to reject that option, it's to make sure you understand what it's doing and what it isn't.

And sometimes, there just isn't a neat answer. You might not know *exactly* why your cycle is irregular. Your labs might come back normal. You might not have a clear cause that fits into a tidy diagnosis. That doesn't mean you're overreacting or that your body's broken. It just means hormones are complex, and sometimes the best care is managing what you can see and feel, not chasing a label.

This scenario is for anyone whose periods have gone rogue and who wants real care, not just a prescription to hide the symptoms. Your cycle may be trying to tell you something. You deserve to be taken seriously, have your options explained, and feel supported in whichever path you choose, whether that includes birth control, lifestyle changes, or further evaluation. What matters most is that you're part of the plan, not just handed one.

Causes of irregular periods:

- **PCOS.** This is a hormonal condition that can cause irregular or absent periods, acne, excess hair growth, and insulin resistance.
- **Thyroid disorders.** Both overactive (hyperthyroidism) and underactive (hypothyroidism) thyroid function can disrupt your cycle.
- **Stress.** Physical or emotional stress can affect ovulation and delay or skip periods.
- **Significant weight changes.** Rapid gain or loss can affect hormonal balance and cycle regularity.
- **Exercise.** Intense training or low body fat can suppress ovulation and lead to missed periods.
- **Eating disorders.** Restrictive eating or nutrient deficiencies can alter reproductive hormones.
- **Perimenopause.** As estrogen levels fluctuate in your 40s (sometimes earlier), cycles may shorten, lengthen, or skip altogether.
- **Medications.** Some antidepressants, antipsychotics, steroids, or blood thinners can affect menstrual patterns. Changing medications can, too.
- **Recent illness or infection.** Acute illness or major changes in your immune system can temporarily disrupt your cycle.
- **Unknown.** Sometimes we just don't know.

What Is PCOS and Why Does It Matter?

Let's start with the basics because PCOS is one of the most common yet most misunderstood hormonal conditions. It affects roughly 1 in 10 people with ovaries during their reproductive years, yet many don't realize they have it or are told they might when they actually don't.

What's Common

PCOS is a hormonal and metabolic condition that can affect your cycles, skin, hair, and overall health. The main features include the following:

- **Irregular or absent periods** (cycles longer than 35 days or fewer than 8 per year)
- **High levels of androgens** (hormones like testosterone that can cause acne, excess hair growth, or hair thinning)
- **Polycystic-appearing ovaries** (ovaries that look enlarged or contain multiple small follicles on ultrasound)

You only need two of these three criteria to be diagnosed. That means you can have PCOS without visible cysts and you can have it even if your weight, skin, or hair look completely typical.

Different Ways PCOS Can Present

For some people, PCOS is a straightforward diagnosis: cycles are irregular or absent, hormone levels are clearly elevated, and ultrasound findings are consistent. These are the classic signs, the kind most clinicians are trained to recognize right away.

But for others, it's not so obvious. You might have mostly regular cycles but struggle with acne, insulin resistance, or fertility changes. You might not have textbook lab results, or your symptoms may overlap with other hormonal or thyroid conditions. In these cases, diagnosis takes more nuance—and sometimes, patience. Not fitting the classic picture doesn't mean your symptoms aren't real. It means your care should be individualized, not one-size-fits-all.

Common Misconceptions

PCOS isn't caused by something you did or didn't do. It's not your fault. It's also not cured by weight loss or a single prescription. While lifestyle changes can help manage symptoms, PCOS is a complex condition influenced by genetics, environment, and hormones. Another myth: PCOS always equals infertility. Not true. Many people with PCOS conceive naturally or with minimal support once their cycles are better understood and managed.

Why It's Often Missed or Misunderstood

Because PCOS looks different from person to person, it's one of the most frequently missed or misdiagnosed reproductive conditions. Irregular periods might get blamed on stress. Weight gain might be chalked up to "bad habits." Or, for those with thinner bodies, the possibility of PCOS might not even be mentioned. On the flip side, some people are told they have PCOS based solely on one irregular cycle or a single ultrasound, when it's really something else. The point: diagnosis should be thoughtful, not rushed or ignored.

What a Diagnosis Actually Means for You

Getting a PCOS diagnosis isn't a dead end. It's a framework for understanding your body. It helps you and your clinician connect the dots with your symptoms, hormone balance, metabolism, and long-term health. Because PCOS is both a reproductive and metabolic condition, it's an opportunity to monitor things like blood sugar, cholesterol, and heart health early on. And once you know what you're working with, you can build a plan that protects your wellbeing now *and* later.

Who Should Be on Your Care Team

Managing PCOS often works best when you have a few people in your corner:

- Your **OB-GYN** can help regulate your cycle, support fertility, and manage reproductive symptoms.
- Your **primary care provider** keeps an eye on your overall health: blood sugar, cholesterol, blood pressure, and long-term monitoring.
- An **endocrinologist** can be especially helpful if your hormone levels are complex or if you have insulin resistance, thyroid conditions, or unusual lab results.

Ideally, these clinicians communicate with each other so your care feels coordinated, not pieced together.

The takeaway: PCOS doesn't look the same for everyone. For some, it's a clear diagnosis; for others, it's a process of connecting subtle dots. Either way, understanding it gives you a powerful tool: insight into how your body works and what it needs.

What to Look for in a Clinician

This isn't about replacing medical care. It's about helping you recognize what *good* care looks like and feel confident being an active partner in it. You don't need to have all the answers walking in. You just deserve a clinician who's curious, collaborative, and willing to dig deeper with you.

When you bring up irregular periods or possible PCOS, the right clinician won't rush to hand you birth control and send you on your way. They'll take the time to understand what's happening in your body, explain the possibilities, and work *with* you to find a plan that fits.

Red Flags: When Care Feels Dismissive or Incomplete

If you hear any of these, it may be time to ask more questions or seek another opinion:

- "Just take birth control to regulate your periods. That'll fix everything."
- "You're too young to worry about PCOS."
- "Lose weight and your periods will become regular."
- "Everyone's cycle is different. Don't worry about it."
- Prescribing hormones without any lab work or explanation.
- Brushing off other symptoms like acne, hair growth, weight changes, or mood shifts as unrelated to your cycle.

Green Lights: Signs You're in Good Hands

A clinician who's truly engaged in your care will do the following:

- Ask about your full symptom picture, not just your periods.
- Order labs and imaging when needed and explain what each test checks for.
- Explore how your thyroid, insulin, stress, and overall health intersect with your cycle.
- Offer multiple treatment paths, not just birth control.
- Acknowledge the impact your symptoms have on your daily life.
- Talk about long-term prevention, monitoring, and emotional well-being.

Tests and evaluations to discuss together. You don't need every test, but knowing what's typically part of an evaluation can help you feel informed and involved in your care. A thorough workup for irregular periods or possible PCOS often includes bloodwork to check hormone balance, thyroid function, and how your body is processing insulin and glucose. Your clinician might also look at cholesterol levels, blood counts, or other markers that offer a fuller picture of your overall health. In some cases, a pelvic ultrasound can help visualize the ovaries and uterus to rule out structural causes of irregular bleeding. The goal isn't to run every test, it's to gather enough information to understand what your body is doing and guide your care plan accordingly.

What collaborative treatment can look like. Treatment for PCOS and irregular periods isn't just about "fixing" your cycle. It's about finding balance, protecting your long-term health, and addressing the symptoms that affect your daily life. A thoughtful clinician will work *with* you to build a plan that might include these supports:

Hormonal management:

- Birth control pills, patches, or IUDs to regulate cycles and protect the uterine lining
- Metformin to improve insulin sensitivity
- Spironolactone to manage acne or excess hair growth

Lifestyle and supportive care:

- Nutrition guidance to stabilize blood sugar (not restrictive diets)
- Regular, moderate exercise
- Stress management and adequate rest
- Mental health and body-image support

Long-term monitoring:

- Routine screening for diabetes, cholesterol, and heart health
- Monitoring bone density if cycles are absent for long stretches
- Revisiting treatment plans as your goals or health needs change

This isn't a checklist to follow on your own, it's a conversation starter. The goal isn't to self-diagnose but to make sure your care feels collaborative, transparent, and grounded in respect.

Pre-Visit Planning

Track your symptoms for at least three months before your visit if possible. This gives your provider a clearer picture of what's happening.

Symptom	Experiencing It? (✓)	How Often/ Severe?	Impact on Life (1 = minimal, 10 = severe)	Notes
Irregular or missing periods				
Very heavy periods				
Severe cramps or pelvic pain				
Acne (especially on face, chest, back)				
Excess hair growth (hirsutism)				
Hair loss or thinning				
Weight gain or difficulty losing weight				
Mood swings or depression				
Fatigue or low energy				
Trouble sleeping				
Skin tags or dark patches (neck, armpits)				

What You Can Ask and How to Prioritize It

There's a lot to cover when it comes to irregular periods and PCOS. Star your must-asks or number them in order of importance so you tackle your biggest concerns first.

Understanding what's happening:

☐ What tests can we do to figure out why my periods are irregular?
☐ Should we test for PCOS, thyroid issues, or other hormonal imbalances?
☐ Can you explain what my hormone levels mean and how they might be affecting my symptoms?
☐ Is an ultrasound necessary to check my ovaries?

PCOS-specific questions:

☐ Do my symptoms suggest PCOS, and what does that diagnosis mean for my health?
☐ How is PCOS connected to insulin resistance and diabetes risk?
☐ What are the long-term health risks I should know about?
☐ How might PCOS affect my ability to get pregnant in the future?

Treatment options:

☐ What are my options besides birth control for regulating my periods?
☐ If I do use birth control, which types are best for PCOS symptoms?
☐ Are there medications that can help with insulin resistance or other PCOS symptoms?
☐ What lifestyle changes might help with my symptoms?

Addressing specific symptoms:

☐ Can we talk about treatments for acne or excess hair growth?
☐ Are there options for managing weight gain or difficulty losing weight?
☐ How can I manage mood symptoms related to hormonal fluctuations?

Fertility and reproductive health:

☐ How do irregular periods affect my fertility?
☐ If I want to get pregnant, what should I know about managing PCOS?
☐ What birth control options work best if I have PCOS?

Long-term monitoring:

☐ What ongoing tests or screenings do I need?
☐ How often should I follow up about these symptoms?
☐ Who should I see for ongoing PCOS management—you, an endocrinologist, or a reproductive specialist?

For Support People

They may be dealing with a complex hormonal condition that affects their entire body, not just their periods. They need someone who understands that PCOS affects energy, mood, weight, fertility, and long-term health—and who won't treat it like a minor inconvenience.

Understanding the whole picture. Learn that PCOS affects more than just periods. Be patient with fatigue, mood changes, or physical symptoms that come with hormonal imbalances.

Long-term perspective. PCOS often requires ongoing management rather than quick fixes. Support their commitment to finding sustainable treatment approaches.

Lifestyle support. If they want to make dietary or exercise changes, be supportive without becoming the "health police" or making them feel monitored.

If you're joining for the visit. Help them advocate for comprehensive evaluation and treatment rather than accepting "just take birth control" as the only solution.

Scenario 10

The Pain They Don't See: Endometriosis and Adenomyosis

How to get past dismissal and into diagnosis—real questions, real scripts, real power

Before You Walk In

Endometriosis and adenomyosis are two of the most misunderstood, underdiagnosed, and dismissed conditions in gynecological care.

Let's break it down:

- **Endometriosis** happens when tissue similar to the lining of the uterus grows in places it shouldn't: outside the uterus, on pelvic organs, the bowel, bladder, ovaries, or even the diaphragm. It causes inflammation, scarring, pain, and often deeply affects fertility and quality of life. But you can't always see it on imaging. The only definitive diagnosis is through surgery. And many providers hesitate to refer for that.

- **Adenomyosis** is when endometrial tissue grows *into* the muscular wall of the uterus itself. It often causes heavy, painful periods and intense cramping. But it's even harder to confirm until after a hysterectomy. Imaging is unreliable. Pain is often dismissed. And treatment is frequently delayed until symptoms become unbearable.

The harm isn't just physical, it's emotional. It's financial. It's years of being told to tough it out. To take a stronger pill. To relax. To stop being so sensitive. Most people who live with these conditions have been disbelieved at some point, often by the very providers who were supposed to help them.

So why are these conditions so often gaslit?

Because the pain isn't always visible. Because periods are still treated like something women are supposed to suffer through. Because when patients say they're in pain, they're too often told it's "normal," "just stress," or "part of being a woman."

This isn't just about pain. It's about being believed.

And it's about getting help *before* the pain starts to take over everything else.

People with endo and adeno may live with these symptoms:

- Severe, stabbing cramps that interrupt school, work, or daily life
- Gastrointestinal (GI) issues and bladder symptoms that mimic irritable bowel syndrome or urinary tract infections
- Painful sex, pelvic floor dysfunction, or pain with bowel movements
- Fatigue, mood changes, and depression from chronic pain
- Fertility challenges or pregnancy loss
- Dozens of appointments without answers
- Being told they're exaggerating, drug-seeking, or too sensitive

On average, it takes *7 to 10 years* to be diagnosed with endometriosis. By that time, the damage isn't just physical. It's psychological. It's systemic. It's years of missed care where it's likely that things have only gotten worse or more painful during this time.

You deserve to be heard before it gets that far.

This scenario helps you organize your symptoms, clarify your goals, and come in prepared—whether you're asking for answers for the first time or trying again after being dismissed.

Pre-Visit Planning

Use this to organize your history, symptoms, and priorities before your appointment.

What is this visit for?

☐ First time bringing this up
☐ Following up on previous concerns
☐ Second opinion
☐ Discuss imaging or labs

☐ Fertility concerns
☐ Period pain or GI symptoms
☐ Something else: _____

What are your top symptoms?

_____
_____
_____

What's your main goal for this visit?

☐ Take me seriously
☐ Get a diagnosis
☐ Get a referral
☐ Get treatment
☐ Ask about surgery or options
☐ Something else: _____

Your Symptom Story

Use the following tracker to capture the full picture. Let's look not just at what's happening, but at how it's affecting your daily life.

Too often, people with conditions like endometriosis or adenomyosis are asked to rate their pain on a scale, without anyone asking how that pain actually shows up in the real world. This tool helps bridge that gap.

You're not just documenting symptoms—you're helping your provider *see* your experience *and* giving yourself a chance to learn from it.

- **What's happening.** When it occurs, where it hurts, how often it shows up
- **How it's affecting you.** Work, relationships, mental health, daily functioning
- **What it's teaching you.** Patterns in your own body, triggers, what helps and what doesn't
- **Why it matters.** This isn't just discomfort—it's information about your body and your life, and it deserves to be understood

Whether this is your first visit or your fifth, this is your opportunity to tell the full story—to your clinician and to yourself. This is your record of what it's like to live in your body, and that story deserves to be taken seriously.

Symptom	Experiencing It? (✓)	How Often? (e.g., daily, weekly)	Impact on Life (1 = minimal, 10 = severe)	Notes
Severe cramping before or during periods				
Pain with bowel movements or urination				
Heavy or prolonged bleeding				
Bleeding through tampons or pads within an hour				
Pain during or after sex				
Chronic pelvic or lower back pain (not just with period)				
Fatigue or exhaustion around your cycle				
Nausea, bloating, or GI symptoms tied to your cycle				

Cycle and Pain Patterns

How many days do you bleed each cycle? _____

Is your pain predictable or random? _____

Do you have pain with:

☐ Ovulation
☐ Sex
☐ Exercise
☐ Defecation (pooping)

Pain Flares and Management

When is it at its worst? _____

How does it interfere with your routine? _____

What have you tried to relieve pain? And what has/hasn't helped? _____

Life Disruption and Mental Health

☐ Missed school/work
☐ Emergency room visits
☐ Cancelled social plans
☐ Sex life or relationship challenges
☐ Anxiety or depression connected to chronic pain

Fertility and Future Concerns

Are you currently trying to get pregnant? _____

Any history of miscarriages or infertility? _____

Do you have concerns about your future options? _____

Other Thoughts

Use this space to jot down anything else you want your provider to know. This might include the following information:

- How long this has been going on
- What support you've had or not had
- Emotional toll, mental health, or relationship impacts
- Why you're seeking answers now

_____

_____

_____

_____

Questions to Ask Your Clinician

Keep in mind: you probably won't have time to ask every question on this list. Prioritize what matters most to you. Put a star next to the ones you don't want to leave without answers, or number them in the order you plan to ask. This helps you stay focused in the moment and ensures the most important concerns get covered.

Getting Clarity on What's Going On

- Based on my symptoms, could this be endometriosis, adenomyosis, or something similar?
- What tests or imaging (like ultrasound or magnetic resonance imaging) can help, and what are their limitations?
- If nothing shows up right away, what's the next step for figuring this out?

Exploring Treatment Options

- What are my options for managing pain and symptoms—both short term and long term?
- Can we start treatment (like hormonal therapy) even without a confirmed diagnosis?
- Are there nonhormonal or lifestyle approaches that could help?
- What are the pros and cons of options like birth control, intrauterine devices (IUDs), or surgery?

Considering Surgery (If Relevant)

- If surgery becomes an option, can you refer me to someone who specializes in excision?
- What's the difference between ablation and excision. How do I know what's right for me?

Navigating Daily Life and Mental Health

- Can you document my symptoms so it's easier to get support at work or school?
- Could I get a note for accommodations, time off, or pain management?
- Can you help me connect with mental health or chronic pain support resources?

If Fertility Is on Your Mind

- How might this condition affect my fertility or ability to get pregnant later?
- If I'm trying to conceive, what should I know about timelines, referrals, or next steps?

For Support People

They're living with chronic pain that's often invisible and too often dismissed. Not just by strangers, but by medical providers, loved ones, even people they've trusted. They need someone who doesn't question what they're feeling. Someone who has their back in a system that still treats pelvic pain as exaggeration, anxiety, or "just part of being a woman."

Believe their pain. Fully, without hesitation. Don't downplay it. Don't ask them to tough it out. Chronic pelvic pain is real. It's complex. And it can be physically and emotionally life-altering.

Help make life more livable. Pain flares can derail even basic routines. Be the person who adjusts without guilt-tripping, whether that means changing plans, covering for them, or just offering grace when they need rest.

Push back with them when they're dismissed. If a provider shrugs it off or suggests it's "just stress," don't stay silent. Support their right to better answers. Help them seek a provider who treats their pain like it matters, because it does.

If you're going with them to a visit. Let them lead, but be ready to back them up. If the provider starts minimizing what they've shared, speak up: "I've seen how bad this gets. This isn't manageable. She deserves a real plan."

Because no one should have to advocate alone while they're in pain.

Scenario 11

When Vaginal or Urinary Symptoms Keep Coming Back

Yeast, BV, UTIs, STI testing, and how to advocate when symptoms keep coming back

Vaginal and urinary symptoms are some of the most common reasons people seek gynecologic care. Burning. Discharge. Odor. Itching. Pelvic discomfort. Urgency. Pain with sex. And yet these are also some of the most frequently dismissed concerns in reproductive healthcare.

Many people are told it's "probably yeast," given a prescription without testing, or reassured that everything looks normal even when symptoms keep coming back. Others are treated repeatedly without anyone stepping back to ask why the problem hasn't resolved.

When something feels off in your body and you're told it's nothing, it can make you doubt your instincts. This scenario is here to help you walk in prepared, understand what may be happening, and leave with a plan instead of another guess.

Understanding What Vaginal and Urinary Symptoms Can Mean

Not all vaginal or urinary symptoms come from the same cause, even when they feel similar. Burning, irritation, discharge, and pelvic discomfort can overlap across multiple conditions, and standard testing does not always capture the full picture.

Common causes include yeast infections, bacterial vaginosis (BV), urinary tract infections (UTIs), sexually transmitted infections (STIs), and inflammatory or microbiome-related conditions. Some resolve easily. Others recur. Some are missed entirely when testing is limited or symptoms don't follow textbook patterns.

Why These Symptoms Are So Often Dismissed

Vaginal and urinary complaints are frequently minimized because they are common, uncomfortable to talk about, and often squeezed into short problem visits. Many clinicians default to empiric treatment, meaning treatment without testing, especially if symptoms sound familiar.

Bias can also creep in. People are judged based on body size, sexual history, relationship status, hygiene myths, or how confidently they describe symptoms. When symptoms recur, patients are sometimes framed as difficult rather than under-evaluated.

None of this means your symptoms aren't real. It means the system often fails to slow down enough to listen.

When "Everything Is Normal" Doesn't Match How You Feel

Hearing that your tests are "normal" can be confusing and deeply invalidating when your body is still uncomfortable or in pain. A normal result does not always mean nothing is wrong. Often, it means that the testing performed was limited, timed in a way that missed what was happening, or designed to look for only a narrow set of causes.

Many routine panels focus on the most common infections, such as yeast or bacterial vaginosis. While those tests are useful, they do not capture every possible explanation for ongoing symptoms. Some infections fluctuate and may not be present at the exact moment a sample is collected. Others can be partially treated or temporarily suppressed, making them harder to detect. Some conditions do not show up on standard testing at all.

In addition, not all vaginal or urinary symptoms are caused by an active infection. Inflammation, changes in the vaginal microbiome, hormone shifts, irritation, or tissue sensitivity can all cause real discomfort even when basic tests are negative. These causes often require a different approach than simply repeating the same medication.

Sometimes the missing question is not just "What is this?" but "Why does this keep happening?" Recurrent symptoms deserve a deeper conversation about patterns, triggers, prior treatments, and what has or has not helped in the past. That context is just as important as the test result itself.

You are allowed to ask what was ruled out, what was not tested for, and what the plan is if symptoms continue. A normal test should be the beginning of a clearer explanation, not the end of the conversation.

When Recurrent Infections Involve a Partner

If you keep being treated for the same infection and it keeps coming back, it's reasonable to wonder whether someone else in the picture might be part of the cycle. That doesn't mean blame. It doesn't mean anyone did anything wrong. It means your body is asking for a different plan.

For a long time, BV was treated as a solo problem. The person with symptoms got medication. Partners were rarely mentioned, evaluated, or included. When BV came back, the answer was often just another round of the same treatment. Many people were left feeling frustrated, embarrassed, or like their body was somehow failing.

That approach is starting to shift.

In 2025, new research showed that treating male partners at the same time as the patient significantly lowered the chances of BV coming back. This mattered because it confirmed something many people already suspected from lived experience. BV-associated bacteria can be shared between partners, even when the other partner has no symptoms at all. Treating just one person may help temporarily, but it may not fully break the cycle.

And this isn't only about male partners.

We've also known for a long time that people with female partners experience BV more often and deal with higher rates of recurrence. That doesn't mean BV is a "sex problem" or that anyone is doing something wrong. It means vaginal environments can influence one another through sex, skin contact, oral-genital contact, shared sex toys, and fluid exchange. Biology is involved, not morality.

The science and guidelines have not caught up equally for all partner configurations, but many clinicians who care for patients with recurrent BV recognize that ignoring partner dynamics altogether often leads to repeat treatment without lasting relief.

Recurrent UTIs and What to Do Next

Recurrent UTIs are exhausting. They hurt, they interrupt daily life, and they're often treated as a nuisance rather than a real quality-of-life issue. Many people are told to drink more water, take another antibiotic, and move on, even when UTIs keep returning. A UTI that comes back is not a personal failure. It's a signal that prevention hasn't been fully addressed yet.

For many people, UTIs are closely linked to sex. That doesn't mean sex is the problem. It means bacteria can be introduced into the urethra during intercourse, especially in people with vulvas and shorter urethras. When UTIs reliably show up after sex, patterns matter, and so do prevention strategies.

One of the simplest and most effective first steps is urinating after intercourse every single time. This helps flush bacteria out of the urethra before they have a chance to travel upward and cause an infection. For some people, this step alone significantly reduces UTIs. For others, it helps but isn't enough. If you're already peeing after sex consistently and infections keep happening, that's important information, not a failure on your part.

When UTIs continue to flare after intercourse despite good hydration and post-sex urination, it's reasonable to shift the conversation from repeated treatment to prevention. One evidence-based option is postcoital antibiotics, which involve taking a single low-dose antibiotic after sex to prevent an infection from developing. For many people with recurrent UTIs, this approach dramatically reduces infections and helps break the cycle. It does not mean you'll be on antibiotics forever. It means using a targeted tool when there is a clear, repeatable trigger.

Sex-related triggers are also allowed to be part of the conversation. Some people notice UTIs flare more often when a partner ejaculates inside the vagina. That doesn't mean semen is dirty or that anyone is doing something wrong. Semen can change the vaginal and urinary environment in ways that make infections more likely for some bodies. If this feels like a trigger for you, it's reasonable to experiment with ejaculation outside the body or barrier use and see whether symptoms improve. These are practical adjustments, not moral judgments.

It's also important to name that not all urinary symptoms are caused by infections. Burning, urgency, or bladder discomfort can persist even when urine cultures are negative or antibiotics don't help. When that happens, repeating the same treatment may not help and can sometimes make things worse. This is often the point where a different kind of evaluation is needed.

If UTIs keep coming back, especially if you're needing antibiotics multiple times a year, this is often when a referral to a urologist makes sense. OB-GYN clinicians manage a lot of urinary issues, but urologists specialize in the bladder, urethra, and urinary tract. They can look more closely at things like bladder function, anatomy, recurrent infection patterns, and whether additional testing or imaging is warranted.

Seeing a urologist doesn't mean something is seriously wrong. It means your symptoms have crossed from an occasional problem into a pattern that deserves deeper evaluation. A urologist may help determine whether infections are truly recurring, whether something else is being mistaken for UTIs, or whether a long-term prevention plan would be safer and more effective than repeated short courses of antibiotics.

If this feels like the right next step, you're allowed to ask for it directly. You can say something as simple as "These UTIs keep coming back. I'd like to be referred to urology to look at prevention and next steps." That's not giving up on your OB-GYN care. It's using the right specialist at the right time.

If UTIs keep returning, the goal isn't just to treat the next infection. It's to stop living in a cycle of pain, antibiotics, and uncertainty. You deserve a plan that reduces how often this happens and helps you feel more in control of your body again.

Testing: What to Ask For and Why It Matters

Testing isn't about proving your symptoms. It's about making sure treatment actually matches what's happening. Testing guides treatment. Without it, people often end up cycling through medications without clarity.

Depending on your symptoms, it's reasonable to ask about the following:

- Vaginal swabs rather than symptom-based treatment
- Urine cultures with antibiotic sensitivity testing instead of urine dipsticks alone
- STI testing that matches your anatomy and sexual practices
- Repeat testing when symptoms persist or recur

Pre-Visit Planning

What is this visit for?

☐ New vaginal or urinary symptoms
☐ Recurrent symptoms

☐ Symptoms not responding to treatment
☐ STI testing
☐ Review of prior results
☐ Second opinion
☐ Something else: _____

What are your top symptoms?

(Write here)

What's your main goal?

☐ Identify the cause of symptoms
☐ Get testing before treatment
☐ Understand why this keeps happening
☐ Review past treatments and results
☐ Get a clear follow-up plan
☐ Address pain or discomfort
☐ Something else: _____

Your Symptom Story

Symptom	Experiencing It? (✓)	How Often?	Impact on Life (1–10)	Notes
Itching or irritation				
Burning (vaginal or urinary)				
Discharge changes				
Odor				
Pelvic discomfort				
Pain with sex				
Urinary urgency or frequency				
Pain with urination				

Patterns and triggers:

When did symptoms start? _____

Do they worsen with sex, your cycle, stress, or antibiotics? _____

What have you tried?

Medications, home remedies, previous diagnoses, and whether they helped or not.

If BV keeps coming back, you are allowed to ask bigger questions:

- Could a partner be contributing to recurrence?
- What does the most up-to-date evidence suggest?
- Would it make sense for both partners to be evaluated or treated?
- Are temporary changes during treatment, like barrier use or pausing shared toys, recommended?

If UTIs keep coming back, you are allowed to ask bigger questions:

- Do my symptoms meet criteria for recurrent UTIs?
- Should we be doing urine cultures and antibiotic sensitivity before treating each episode?
- Would postcoital antibiotics or another prevention strategy make sense for me?
- At what point should I be referred to urology for further evaluation?
- If cultures are negative, what else could be causing these symptoms?
- What is the plan if this keeps happening over the next few months?

For Support People

Vaginal and urinary symptoms can be physically uncomfortable and emotionally isolating. They're often minimized, joked about, or treated as embarrassing. What helps most is simple belief

Listen without trying to fix. Validate that recurring symptoms are exhausting and frustrating. Help them keep track of patterns or attend appointments if they ask. And remind them that needing answers doesn't mean they're doing anything wrong. It means their body is asking for care.

Scenario 12

Ovarian Cysts, Scary Pain, and Real Answers

Understanding the types of cysts, what symptoms matter, and how to build a follow-up plan that actually protects your peace

Before You Walk In

Ovarian cysts are incredibly common. Most are harmless and temporary. But that doesn't make them any less stressful when you're the one in pain, doubled over in the middle of the night, or staring at an ultrasound report with words no one bothered to explain.

Understanding the Different Types of Ovarian Cysts

Most ovarian cysts are benign and go away on their own. But not all cysts behave the same way, and knowing the differences can help you feel more grounded when an ultrasound suddenly becomes part of your life.

Some cysts need only time and repeat imaging. Some need pain management. Some need monitoring. Some need surgery. And you deserve to know which category you fall into—not assume, not guess, and not feel brushed aside.

Functional Cysts

Functional cysts are the most common and often the least dramatic, even if they're the ones that cause the most stress when you hear the word *cyst*. These form from your normal menstrual cycle and often appear as "simple" cysts: thin-walled, fluid-filled, and completely benign-looking.

They usually cause no symptoms and often disappear on their own within six to eight weeks. Many clinicians reassure that they're "normal." But they can still cause pressure, bloating, or pain. Most of the time, they just need time and a follow-up ultrasound.

Some simple cysts can be 4, 5, even 6 to 8 cm without being dangerous. Larger simple cysts may not disappear as quickly as smaller ones, but they're still benign-appearing and often managed with watchful waiting unless they become painful or keep growing.

Cystadenomas

Cystadenomas form on the outer surface of the ovary. They're benign but can grow quite large, which is usually why they cause discomfort. These do not resolve on their own. Even though they aren't cancerous, their size alone can make surgery the right option.

Endometriomas

Endometriomas form because of endometriosis. They don't disappear and often linger or grow over time. They commonly cause pelvic pain or pain during certain activities. Management depends on symptoms and life plans, especially related to fertility.

Teratomas (Dermoid Cysts)

Teratomas are benign tumors that contain different types of tissue, like skin or hair. They don't go away on their own and may need to be removed if they get large or cause symptoms. They are almost always benign.

Cysts Behave Differently in Every Body

Some people walk around with cysts for months and never know they're there. Others end up in the emergency room (ER) with pain so sharp it takes their breath away.

Many only learn they had a cyst after it bursts. And sometimes a cyst that looked small and harmless on ultrasound ends up being the source of weeks of unexplained discomfort.

That's why blanket reassurance can feel invalidating. Your experience might not be "mild." Your pain might not be "normal." Your body might not match what the textbook says.

Why Cysts Are Often Dismissed

Cysts are common, and many resolve on their own. Because of that, pelvic pain is often minimized before your symptoms are even discussed. And cyst pain doesn't behave predictably. It can be a dull ache or a stabbing shock. It can radiate into your back, pelvis, or vagina. It can worsen with movement, sex, a full bladder, or sometimes for no clear reason at all.

For many people, the pain only becomes obvious when something changes inside the cyst, like when it ruptures.

A rupture can cause sudden, severe pain that makes you double over, sweat, or vomit. It can feel like something popped or tore inside your pelvis. Sometimes the pain tapers on its own; other times you need medical care. Larger cysts are more likely to rupture.

Another possible complication is ovarian torsion. It's uncommon, but it happens. Torsion occurs when a cyst grows large enough to pull the ovary out of position, causing it to twist and cut off blood flow. The pain is intense, escalating, and often paired with nausea or vomiting. Torsion is a medical emergency requiring prompt evaluation and often surgical treatment.

You deserve good care. This scenario helps you walk in prepared: clarifying your symptoms, understanding the questions that matter, and having scripts for when you need clearer answers or firmer guidance. Your fear deserves clarity. Your pain deserves evaluation. And your body deserves a plan that makes sense.

How Cyst Pain Can Mimic Other Abdominal Emergencies

Pelvic pain can be confusing. Ovarian cyst pain can feel exactly like appendicitis, kidney stones, diverticulitis, or other gastrointestinal (GI) issues. It often shows up as sharp pain on the lower right or left side of the abdomen, sometimes higher than expected, and may come with nausea or vomiting. Because of this, some people are first evaluated for stomach or bowel problems before anyone considers their ovaries.

That overlap can delay the right imaging or lead to pain being brushed off as "just GI." Both approaches matter. You deserve a work-up that checks the abdomen *and* the pelvis when symptoms fit either picture.

Imaging: What to Ask for and When to Repeat It

Ultrasound is the main tool clinicians use to understand ovarian cysts. It shows where the cyst is, what it looks like, how big it is, and whether it's filled with clear fluid or something more complex.

In some situations, especially in the ER, a CT scan may be ordered to rule out other urgent causes of abdominal or pelvic pain, such as appendicitis, kidney stones, or bowel issues. While CT scans can sometimes identify ovarian cysts, they are not as precise as ultrasound for evaluating ovarian structures and cyst characteristics.

If you're in the ER and a CT scan is performed, it's reasonable to ask whether a pelvic ultrasound is still needed for follow-up, particularly if ovarian pain or a cyst is suspected.

When to Get Imaging

Ask for an ultrasound if you have any of these symptoms:

- New pelvic pain
- One-sided pain that keeps returning
- A known cyst and changing symptoms
- A suspected rupture (follow-up only)
- Fertility concerns
- A prior cyst and want to know if it's still there

Most cysts are evaluated with a transvaginal ultrasound, but abdominal ultrasound can be used based on comfort and anatomy.

When to Repeat Imaging

Repeat ultrasounds are usually recommended in these situations:

- A cyst is larger than 4–5 cm.
- A simple cyst is sizable (6–7 cm).
- The cyst doesn't clearly look functional.
- Symptoms aren't improving.
- The clinician wants to confirm the cyst is shrinking.

Typical follow-up timing:

- 6–12 weeks for functional/simple cysts
- 3 months for borderline or unclear cysts
- Sooner if symptoms escalate or change suddenly

When to Go to the ER: When Pain Is Sudden, Severe, or Just Feels "Wrong"

Most cysts never lead to emergencies. But when pelvic pain shifts suddenly, becoming sharp, severe, or completely out of character, it's important to get evaluated.

These symptoms don't always mean something dangerous is happening, but they are strong signals your body needs timely medical attention.

Go to the ER if you experience any of these symptoms:

- Sudden, intense pelvic or abdominal pain
- Pain with dizziness, faintness, or weakness
- Pain with nausea or vomiting that doesn't ease
- Pain so strong you can't stand, walk, or breathe normally
- Unexpected new vaginal bleeding
- Severe right- or left-sided lower abdominal pain that feels like appendicitis or a stomach emergency

Why Being Seen Matters

The goal isn't just to check the cyst. It's to rule out what we do not want to miss:

- **Ovarian torsion.** Sudden severe pain always warrants ruling out torsion.
- **Ectopic pregnancy.** Even if you don't think you're pregnant, this must be ruled out because an ectopic can mimic a cyst rupture or appendicitis and may escalate quickly.

Neither torsion nor ectopic pregnancy is common, but both matter enough that you should never hesitate to be seen.

Bottom line. If something feels suddenly wrong, see a clinician.

You are not overreacting and quick action can be important.

When Surgery Becomes Part of the Discussion

Surgery is considered when the goal is to prevent repeat pain, manage something that won't resolve on its own, or reduce the risk of future complications. This is almost always a planned, not emergency, pathway—meaning you get time to ask questions, weigh options, and meet with the right clinician.

Surgery may enter the conversation if any of the following occurs:

- The cyst is large (often above 5–7 cm).
- The cyst type is one that doesn't go away on its own (like dermoids, cystadenomas, endometriomas).
- Pain is persistent even after the acute episode passes.
- Follow-up imaging shows the cyst isn't shrinking or is growing.
- There was concern for torsion and your ovary looks compromised on imaging.
- Symptoms keep sending you back to urgent care or the ER.
- You want a definitive solution rather than ongoing monitoring.

None of these mean surgery is required, only that it can be reasonable to discuss.

This is also when it matters *whom* you talk to. Ovarian cyst surgery should be discussed with a doctor who does these procedures regularly and can explain the benefits, risks, and impact on fertility in plain language.

You are not signing up for anything by having this conversation.
You're gathering information. You're asking what's possible.
You're making sure the next steps match your body, your goals, and your life.

Pre-Visit Planning

Use this section to organize what's happening in your body, what you're worried about, and what you want from this appointment.

What is this visit for?

☐ First time bringing this up
☐ Review an ultrasound
☐ New or worsening pelvic pain
☐ Suspected rupture
☐ Second opinion
☐ Fertility concerns
☐ Discussing surgical options
☐ Something else: _____

What are your top symptoms?
(write here)

_____

_____

What's your main goal?
☐ Understand what type of cyst this is
☐ Have my symptoms taken seriously
☐ Go over imaging in plain language
☐ Get a monitoring or follow-up plan
☐ Learn about pain management
☐ Clarify when to worry or go to the ER
☐ Explore whether surgery is appropriate
☐ Something else: _____

Your Symptom Story

This is where you capture the full picture of your experience, not just the pain, but how it shows up in your life. Many people with ovarian cysts are told "everything looks fine" even when they're in significant discomfort. This helps bridge that gap.

Symptom	Experiencing It? (✓)	How Often?	Impact on Life (1–10)	Notes
One-sided pelvic pain				
Pressure or fullness				
Sharp or sudden pain				
Bloating or distention				
Pain during or after sex				
Pain with movement				
Nausea or vomiting with pain				
Pain around ovulation				
Feeling of "tugging" or heaviness				

Patterns and triggers:

Where in your body do you feel the pain? _____

When do symptoms usually show up? _____

Do you have pain with:

- ☐ Ovulation
- ☐ Sex
- ☐ Exercise
- ☐ Bowel movements
- ☐ A full bladder
- ☐ Sudden movements
- ☐ Other

Pain flares and management:

When is it at its worst?

_____

_____

How does it interfere with daily life?

_____

_____

What have you tried—and what has or hasn't helped?

_____

_____

Imaging: What you want to clarify:
Imaging is often the key to understanding cysts, but only if someone explains what was seen and what it means for you. Use this section to guide your questions.

Do I need imaging today?

- ☐ Yes
- ☐ No
- ☐ I'm not sure — I want to ask

If I already had imaging, I want to understand the following:

- ☐ What type of cyst it looks like
- ☐ Whether it's simple or complex

- [ ] The size and how size matters
- [ ] Whether it could resolve on its own
- [ ] Whether I need a repeat ultrasound
- [ ] What changes would be concerning

Questions for your clinician:

- "What type of cyst is this?"
- "When should I repeat imaging?"
- "What would you expect this cyst to do over the next 6–12 weeks?"
- "At what point would we change the plan?"

Fertility and future concerns:

Are you trying to get pregnant?

_____

_____

Any history of infertility or miscarriage?

_____

_____

Do you have concerns about how this cyst affects future fertility?

_____

_____

If you want to discuss surgery. Not all cysts require surgery. But if yours is large, persistent, painful, or not the kind that resolves on its own, it's reasonable to talk about it.

What you may want to ask:

- "What size or symptoms would make surgery the safer option?"
- "Do you perform this type of surgery often?"
- "Would minimally invasive surgery be possible?"
- "How would surgery affect my fertility?"
- "Should I see a surgeon who specializes in ovarian surgery?"

Other thoughts:

Anything else on your mind: fears, expectations, patterns you've noticed, things you're hoping for:

_____

_____

For Support People

Pelvic pain from ovarian cysts can be confusing, unpredictable, and often invisible. One day they may feel mostly fine; the next, a simple movement can send pain shooting through their pelvis. What makes this even harder is that cyst pain is frequently minimized by clinicians, by friends, by family. They need someone who believes them without hesitation.

Believe their pain—completely. Don't assume that because a cyst is "small" on an ultrasound, the pain must be small, too. Size doesn't always match severity, and ruptures or pressure changes can hurt intensely. Trust what they're telling you about their body.

Stay flexible when symptoms flare. Cyst pain can interrupt plans with no warning. Be the person who doesn't guilt-trip, sigh, or make them feel like an inconvenience. Offer comfort, practical help, and the space to rest if that's what their body needs.

Help them feel less alone in a system that often dismisses pelvic pain. If they come out of an appointment feeling brushed off or confused, listen first. Validate what happened. Help them think through next steps, whether that's getting clearer answers, scheduling follow-up imaging, or seeking a second opinion.

If you're going with them to a visit. Let them lead the conversation—it's their body and their story. But if you notice their symptoms being minimized or overlooked, your voice can matter. You might say something like, "I've seen how much pain this causes. It's affecting daily life. We need a plan that actually addresses it."

Your presence can make all the difference. Ovarian cysts can bring uncertainty, fear, and sudden pain. Knowing someone is in it with them—steady, supportive, and believing—can turn a frightening experience into one that feels navigable and held.

Scenario 13

Menopause Misinformation, Hormone Therapy, and Being Taken Seriously

What to track, how to push past the "just aging" line, and the treatment options you deserve

W̲e don't talk about menopause enough, despite the fact that *every woman* will go through it at some point in her life. Half the population will experience this transition, yet most of us were never really taught what it means, how it starts, or what it feels like. And when we finally do start asking questions, we're often met with shrugs, myths, or dismissal.

So let's start with the basics.

Menopause is officially defined as the point when you've gone 12 consecutive months without a menstrual period due to the natural decline in reproductive hormones. If you hit 10 months and then bleed again, the clock resets. The average age of menopause in the United States is about 51, but it can happen earlier or later depending on genetics, medical conditions, or surgeries such as oopharectomy (ovary removal).

Perimenopause is the transition that leads up to menopause. It can begin in your late 30s or early 40s and last for several years. During this time, your ovaries still function, but not consistently. Hormones fluctuate unpredictably. Periods become irregular. And symptoms can feel all over the place. Some months, you're fine. Other months, you're sweating through the sheets, crying in meetings, and forgetting what you walked into the room for.

You're not imagining it. And you're likely not "too young" to be going through it.

When people say they're "going through menopause," they're usually talking about this entire arc: the rollercoaster of perimenopause, the milestone of menopause, and the years of postmenopause that follow. It's not just about your period stopping, it's your whole system recalibrating.

And yet, most healthcare providers still don't take it seriously. They don't screen for it. They don't explain it. They don't offer real treatment options unless you push. Too many women are told it's "just aging" or "normal," as if exhaustion, weight gain, brain fog, and night sweats are simply the price of getting older. But just because something is *common* doesn't mean it's *fine*.

Perimenopause and menopause are major hormonal shifts that affect everything from your mood and sleep to your metabolism, heart health, and bone density. They deserve attention, explanation, and support. Not silence.

You're not crazy. You're not overreacting. You deserve real answers, evidence-based care, and a provider who recognizes that this is not "just part of aging"—it's a fundamental part of health.

Menopause Hormone Therapy (MHT): Sorting Truth from Fear

Menopause hormone therapy (MHT), often referred to as hormone replacement therapy, or HRT, is one of the most effective tools we have for managing menopause symptoms. Yet most people never receive a clear, balanced conversation about it. Instead, they are left with half-truths, outdated fears, or quick dismissals that make it feel like wanting relief is somehow risky or vain.

Much of that confusion traces back more than 20 years to the Women's Health Initiative (WHI), a large 2002 study that fundamentally changed the trajectory of menopause care. Headlines at the time linked hormone therapy to increased risks of breast cancer and heart disease, and the Food and Drug Administration responded by placing a black box warning, its strongest caution label, on estrogen-containing therapies. Prescribing rates dropped sharply almost overnight. What was lost in the fallout was critical context.

The highest risks identified in the WHI were associated with one specific regimen: oral estrogen combined with a synthetic progestin, medroxyprogesterone acetate. These formulations are no longer the standard of care. In addition, the women enrolled in the study were, on average, older and well past the menopausal transition, many starting therapy a decade or more after menopause. Subsequent research has shown that timing matters. Initiating MHT earlier, generally within about 10 years of menopause or before age 60, appears to carry a more favorable risk profile and may offer benefits for heart and brain health for some patients.

In fact, newer evidence paints a far more nuanced picture:

- **Transdermal estradiol** (delivered through a patch, gel, or spray) is both safe and effective for many people who begin treatment near menopause.
- **Micronized progesterone**—a bioidentical form of progesterone—appears to carry fewer clotting and breast cancer risks than older synthetic progestins.
- **Vaginal estrogen** (in creams, rings, or tablets) can treat dryness, pain with sex, and urinary symptoms with almost no systemic absorption or risk.
- And contrary to old rules, there's **no evidence-based age limit** that says HRT must stop at 65. Duration should be individualized, based on symptoms, health profile, and personal comfort.

In 2025, the FDA officially removed the black box warning from hormone replacement therapy, acknowledging that the science had evolved. Yet myths still persist. Many providers were trained during the WHI era and never retrained afterward. Others simply don't feel confident prescribing HRT or discussing options, so patients are told to "tough it out" or handed antidepressants when hormones might have been the appropriate first step. It's not malice, it's a *training gap*. Most medical schools still devote less than a single day to menopause management, and in a healthcare system that rewards volume over conversation, meaningful, nuanced care falls through the cracks.

This isn't a debate, it's a call for better information and better training.

Menopause care shouldn't depend on which provider you happen to see or whether they've kept up with the latest research. Every clinician who cares for people with ovaries should understand the basics of hormone therapy, its risks and benefits, and how to individualize it. Every patient deserves a conversation grounded in current evidence, not outdated fear mongering.

Who Can Benefit Most from Hormone Therapy (and What It Can Do)

Who benefits most:

- **Perimenopause (late 30s–mid 40s).** Can help stabilize hormonal swings causing hot flashes, night sweats, brain fog, and sleep disruption
- **Early menopause (before 45).** Strongly recommended unless contraindicated—protects bone, brain, and heart health from years of hormone loss

- **Typical menopause (around age 51).** The most common time to start; safe and effective for healthy women in their 40s and 50s with moderate or severe symptoms
- **Postmenopause (60s and beyond).** Starting MHT for the first time after 60 carries higher risks, but continuing earlier therapy can remain safe and beneficial
- **At any age.** Can safely treat dryness, pain, or urinary symptoms for nearly everyone, including those who can't take systemic hormones

What hormone therapy can do:

- Reduce hot flashes and night sweats.
- Improve vaginal dryness and discomfort during sex.
- Lower the risk of recurrent urinary infections.
- Support bone health and reduce osteoporosis risk.
- Improve sleep, mood, and energy.
- Help maintain skin hydration and healing.

What it doesn't do:

- Erase every symptom.
- Guarantee protection from heart disease or dementia.
- Work the same way for everyone. Timing, dose, and delivery matter.

Bottom line. You don't need hormone therapy to survive menopause. But you do deserve an informed, evidence-based conversation about it. Being told "there's no point" or "it's too risky" without real discussion isn't care, it's dismissal.

Advocacy Scripts

If you're considering hormone therapy:

- "I'd like to talk about hormone therapy and whether it could help with my symptoms. Can you explain my options?"
- "I understand there are different forms: patches, pills, and creams. Can you tell me how they compare?"
- "If I need progesterone, can we talk about micronized progesterone versus synthetic progestins?"
- "What parts of my history, like blood clots, cancers, or surgeries, make hormone therapy a better or worse fit for me?"

If you're told no:

- "Can you explain why you don't recommend hormone therapy for me specifically, based on my history?"
- "Are there lower-dose or local options that might still be safe?"
- "If you don't prescribe MHT, can you refer me to someone who does?"

Beyond Hot Flashes: How Menopause Affects the Whole Body

Menopause isn't just about hot flashes and mood swings. Estrogen affects nearly every system in the body, including muscles, joints, and connective tissue. As estrogen levels drop, inflammation can increase and collagen production declines. That can show up as stiff joints, slower recovery, or even frozen shoulder (adhesive capsulitis)—a painful condition that limits movement.

It's most common in women between 40 and 60 and often overlaps with perimenopause or early menopause. If you've developed shoulder pain or stiffness, mention it to your clinician. Treatment can include physical therapy, anti-inflammatory medications, or corticosteroid injections. Hormonal changes truly can affect the musculoskeletal system, acknowledging that early can help you get relief faster instead of being brushed off as "just aging."

Common Symptoms to Track

This chart isn't just a checklist. It's a way to spot patterns and give your provider something concrete to respond to. Tracking how often symptoms show up and how much they affect your life turns vague frustration into clear, actionable information.

It helps in two key ways:

- **It validates your experience.** You don't have to remember everything in the moment. You have the details right in front of you.
- **It guides your care.** Certain symptoms or severity levels can shape what your provider recommends and what options are safest or most effective for you.

You don't need to have every symptom or rate everything a 10. The goal is simply to paint a clearer picture so you can walk in and say, "Here's what I've been noticing. Here's how it's affecting me. What are my options?"

In the Notes section, add brief context to bring symptoms to life—when they happen, what you've tried, patterns you've noticed, or how they affect your daily life or relationships. Those details turn numbers into a story and that story helps your provider move from generic advice to care that actually fits you.

Symptom	Experiencing It? (✓)	How Often? (e.g., daily, weekly)	Impact on Life (1 = minimal, 10 = severe)	Notes
Hot flashes or night sweats				
Mood swings, anxiety, or depression				
Insomnia or poor sleep				
Brain fog or trouble concentrating				
Forgetfulness				
Changes in libido				
Vaginal dryness or pain during sex				
Urinary incontinence / increased urinary urgency				
GI changes / constipation				
Weight changes or slowed metabolism				
Joint pain or body aches				
Irregular periods or cycle changes				

Pre-Visit Planning

If you're dealing with hormonal symptoms, this deserves its own dedicated visit. Don't try to squeeze it into your annual exam, you won't get what you need. Annuals are quick, checklist-style visits meant for screenings, not deep conversations about brain fog, night sweats, or why you suddenly feel like a stranger in your own body.

Ask for a separate appointment specifically for perimenopause or hormonal concerns. You deserve focused time and a provider who isn't rushing through your questions. When you schedule a dedicated visit, it signals that this conversation matters. And it gives your clinician the space to actually dive in, instead of treating it like an "oh, by the way" at the end of your Pap smear.

Once that visit is on the calendar, take a few minutes to prepare. There's a lot to cover, and you probably won't get through every question in one sitting—and that's completely okay. The goal is to leave with the information that matters most to *you*.

Mark your must-asks, the questions you absolutely want answered, so you can focus the appointment on your top priorities.

What You Can Ask and How to Prioritize It

Understanding your transition:

- ☐ Can you confirm if I'm in perimenopause? Or is this diagnosis based on symptoms?
- ☐ What changes are expected, and what would warrant more evaluation?
- ☐ Can you explain what's happening hormonally right now?

Hormone therapy and treatment options:

- ☐ What are the risks and benefits of hormone therapy for me specifically?
- ☐ Are there different forms (patch, pill, cream, gel) that might work better for my symptoms or preferences?
- ☐ What are my nonhormonal options, and how effective are they?

Bone, brain, and heart health:

- ☐ Should I be screened for osteoporosis or have a bone density test?
- ☐ How does this transition affect my cardiovascular health?
- ☐ Is there a connection between menopause and memory changes or brain fog?

Sexual health:

- ☐ Can we talk about vaginal dryness, painful sex, or low libido?
- ☐ What treatments actually help? And which are safe for me long term?

Mental health:

☐ Could my mood changes, anxiety, or irritability be hormonal?

☐ Should I see a therapist, or can we address this as part of my menopause care?

Lifestyle strategies:

☐ Are there evidence-based lifestyle changes (nutrition, exercise, sleep, stress) that make a difference?

☐ How much does stress affect symptoms? And how can I manage it?

Ongoing care:

☐ How often should I follow up or reevaluate treatment?

☐ What should I track at home between visits?

☐ If this isn't your area of expertise, who should I see for specialized menopause care?

By walking in with a few priorities circled and your top symptoms noted, you shift the tone of the visit from rushed to intentional. You're showing up informed and organized, which helps your provider show up ready to listen. This isn't about getting through a checklist; it's about making space for a real conversation about your body, your choices, and your next steps.

For Support People

They're navigating a major hormonal shift that affects their body, mind, emotions, and sense of self. All while being told to "just power through." They need someone who takes their experience seriously and supports them through it with care, curiosity, and compassion.

Understand the full scope. Hormonal shifts affect sleep, mood, libido, cognition, and more. These changes are not about "attitude," they're about biology.

Be flexible and patient. Their energy may vary. Intimacy might feel different. Brain fog might make things harder to communicate. Try not to take it personally, this is temporary, and they're adjusting, too.

Reject ageist minimization. Don't brush it off as "just getting older." Support their right to real care, not just platitudes.

If you're joining for the visit. Help them advocate. If the provider starts dismissing their symptoms, reinforce what they've shared: "This has been affecting her daily life. We're hoping for options, not just explanations."

SEX, FERTILITY, AND FAMILY BUILDING

Scenario 14

Sexual Health Beyond "Just Use Lube"

When your sexual wellness needs real care, not dismissive one-liners

♬ Let's talk about sex baby. But for real. Let's talk about the kind of conversation too many people never get to have in the exam room. The most common sexual health questions patients bring to their OB-GYNs usually fall into two categories: "Why does sex hurt?" and "Why don't I want it anymore?" Others ask about trouble reaching orgasm, changes in sensation or desire after giving birth, starting a new birth control, or going through hormone therapy. Some just want to know what's happening to their body and is it normal?

What happens too often in the exam room, is dismissal. Patients are told it's "just stress," or "just aging," or that they should "just use lube." Instead of getting real answers or an actual plan, they leave the office with nothing but a brush-off and a lingering sense that maybe they were foolish for even bringing it up. That's not just inadequate care; it's a missed opportunity to treat a vital part of health and well-being. Sexual health isn't extra. It's not a luxury. It's part of your whole-body care and it deserves more.

And yet, these conversations can feel vulnerable, awkward, or even shame-inducing. But they shouldn't. There's no such thing as TMI, or too much information, with your provider. They're the professional in the room. The one who should make it feel clinical, not shameful. If talking about sex feels hard, remember: this is part of their job. They've heard it all. And if they act uncomfortable, dismissive, or judgmental? That says more about their training gaps and their personal beliefs and stigmas than about you.

You deserve to feel comfortable saying exactly what's happening. Whether that's dryness, pain, loss of desire, or changes after childbirth, birth control, or menopause. When you bring it up, use clear language and describe what it feels like (burning, pressure, loss of sensation, etc.). That helps your clinician understand what's going on, what to evaluate next, and how to help you.

What's Normal?

Here's the truth: there's no single definition of "normal" when it comes to sex or desire. Every body, and every season of life, is different. What's normal for you at 25 is likely to look completely different at 35, 45, and 55, during postpartum, or during perimenopause.

Desire isn't linear. It can fluctuate with stress, sleep, relationship dynamics, hormones, mental health, medications, or even whether you feel emotionally safe and connected. The same goes for orgasm, lubrication, and arousal. They're influenced by your brain just as much as your body.

What's not normal is suffering in silence. Pain, dryness, burning, or bleeding with sex are never things you just have to "push through." Neither is feeling disconnected from your own body or desire. Those are signals, not failures. They're clues that something deserves attention, not proof that you're broken.

And remember: low desire alone isn't automatically a problem. The real question is whether it *bothers* you. If you're content with your sex life, that's what matters. There's no "right" frequency or standard to live up to. But if something feels off, or you want things to be different, you deserve support, not judgment.

Pleasure Is Part of the Picture

Sexual wellness isn't just about pain or dysfunction. It's also about pleasure. You're allowed to want sex to feel good, not just tolerable. And there are real tools, practices, and conversations that can help.

Sexual devices and stimulation tools:

Sex toys can enhance pleasure, support arousal, or even help retrain pelvic floor and vaginal muscles after trauma, childbirth, or hormonal changes.

Vibrators and dilators can help with arousal, blood flow, or penetration-related discomfort.

Couples' toys can strengthen intimacy and communication.

Pelvic wands or massagers may be recommended by pelvic floor physical therapists for pain or muscle tightness.

Safety and sanitation matter:

Use body-safe, nonporous materials (like silicone or stainless steel).

Clean toys after every use with warm water and gentle, fragrance-free soap.

If sharing, use condoms on toys or avoid sharing unless properly sanitized.

Avoid oil-based lubricants with silicone toys. They can break down the material.

Erotica, audio, or visual stimulation:

Smut books deserve a special callout. Romance novels, spicy fiction, and unapologetic smut are changing the conversation about desire because they center internal experience, not performance. They give people permission to feel turned on without being watched, judged, or rushed. You control the pace. You pause when you want. You imagine bodies that feel familiar, aspirational, or entirely fantastical. For many people, especially women, parents, and anyone burned out by real-life expectations, smut works because it reconnects arousal to safety, agency, and emotional context. It is not about visuals or comparison. It is about desire starting in the brain, where it actually lives.

Erotica, guided fantasy, ethical porn, and smut can all help reignite desire and curiosity without pressure to perform. Look for platforms and creators that prioritize consent, representation, and diverse bodies. This can be a solo exploration or something shared with a partner, whatever feels right for you.

The goal is not to fix you. It is to help you reconnect with your body, your pleasure, and your sense of self on your own terms. Sex and desire change throughout your life. That does not mean you are broken. It means you are human. With the right conversations, tools, and care, you can rewrite what intimacy looks like for you, without shame, without comparison, and without apology.

What to Expect from Your Clinician

If you bring up sex, pain, or low desire in the exam room, you deserve a clinician who treats it as real and important, not awkward or optional. Sexual health is a legitimate part of medical care, and a good provider should make space for that conversation instead of brushing it off.

A supportive clinician will take your concerns seriously and ask thoughtful follow-up questions about timing, context, and how your symptoms affects your daily life. They'll look beyond surface-level explanations and consider the full picture: hormones, medications, stress, relationship dynamics, pelvic floor health, and mental well-being. They'll explain possible causes in clear, judgment-free language, outline real treatment options, and collaborate with you to find what feels right for your goals and body. And if they don't have all the answers, they'll refer you to someone who does, like a pelvic floor physical therapist, a sex therapist, or a hormone specialist.

You should leave that appointment feeling heard, informed, and with a plan. Not dismissed, embarrassed, or confused.

Red flags to watch for:

- Dismissing your concerns as "just stress" or "normal aging"
- Making assumptions about your gender, sexuality, or relationship
- Offering only surface-level advice like "try lube" without investigating why you need it
- Ignoring possible hormonal or medical causes
- Rushing the conversation or visibly uncomfortable discussing sex

If you walk out of an appointment feeling small or unseen, that's not a reflection of you, it's a reflection of a training gap in them. The right clinician won't make you feel like a problem; they'll help you solve one.

What Good Care Can Look Like

When a clinician approaches this the right way, the conversation goes deeper than "use more lubricant." They'll talk through hormonal, emotional, and physical contributors—and help you find interventions that match your life.

Hormonal approaches:

- **Topical estrogen** to support vaginal and vulvar tissue health, especially for dryness, pain, or recurrent urinary infections

- **Testosterone therapy** (off-label but evidence-based for women) for low libido or loss of sensation
- **Adjusting or changing birth control methods** if they're affecting desire or comfort

Nonhormonal options:

- **Pelvic floor physical therapy** to address tightness, pain, or muscle tension
- **Medication adjustments,** like switching antidepressants that affect sexual function
- **Nonhormonal medications** for low libido (such as flibanserin or bremelanotide) when appropriate

Therapeutic and behavioral support:

- **Sex therapy** (solo or couples) to improve communication, confidence, and connection
- **Individual therapy** for anxiety, trauma, or relationship stress that may affect intimacy
- **Support groups** for postpartum, menopause, or identity-specific experiences

The best care doesn't reduce this conversation to a hormone level or a pain scale. It acknowledges that sexuality is physical, emotional, relational, and deeply personal. Good care explores all of that, without shame, without assumptions, and without making you feel rushed out of the room.

A Final Note on Sexual Wellness

Sexual health *is* health. Full stop.

Your desire, your comfort, your pleasure. These aren't extras. They're not vanity issues. They're not "too much." They're part of your well-being, and they deserve care.

When something changes, you don't have to just live with it. You don't need to suffer quietly, minimize your experience, or convince yourself it doesn't matter. If your provider can't have this conversation with both knowledge and compassion, find someone who can.

There are clinicians who take sexual wellness seriously. Ones who understand that intimacy, comfort, and connection are essential parts of your overall health.

Your sexual wellness matters.

Your comfort matters.

You matter.

Pre-Visit Planning

What is this visit for?

☐ Decreased libido or sex drive
☐ Difficulty with arousal or orgasm
☐ Sexual changes after birth control, pregnancy, or menopause
☐ LGBTQ+ specific sexual health needs
☐ Relationship/communication concerns
☐ Something else: _____

What's changed for me?

When did I first notice this change? _____

What was different before? _____

Is this affecting my life or relationships?

☐ Yes, significantly
☐ Yes, somewhat
☐ Not yet, but I'm concerned
☐ I just want to understand what's normal

What's Worth Sharing: Context That Helps

Sexual health doesn't exist in a vacuum. It's shaped by the following factors:

- Hormones
- Mental health
- Relationships
- Life stress
- Medications
- Sleep and energy

Context you can share:

- Recent medications (e.g., antidepressants, antihistamines, blood pressure meds)
- Hormonal shifts (birth control, pregnancy, menopause)
- Major stressors (work, caregiving, grief, relationship stress)

- Mental health changes
- Relationship dynamics or communication changes

Helpful self-reflection:

- Is this issue always present, or situational?
- Do I still have desire but struggle with response?
- Has anything helped, even a little?
- Do I want treatment or just answers?

What to Ask in the Exam Room:

Asking the right open ended questions is so helpful when it comes to your sexual health and wellness.

Understanding what's happening:

- "Could this be related to hormonal changes?"
- "Can medications affect sexual function?"
- "Is this something you see often in your patients?"
- "What are common causes of what I'm experiencing?"

Treatment and options:

- "What are my treatment options?"
- "Can hormone therapy help with sexual function?"
- "Would you recommend any specialists—like a sex therapist, hormone specialist, or pelvic physical therapist?"
- "Are there medications that help or ones to avoid?"

Holistic care:

- "How can I talk about this with my partner?"
- "What resources exist for couples dealing with sexual changes?"
- "How do stress, sleep, and mental health affect this?"

For Support People

Sexual health issues don't exist in a vacuum. They can affect relationships, self-esteem, and emotional well-being. And while these concerns are common, they're too often dismissed as "just aging," "just stress," or "just relationship problems" rather than recognized as valid medical concerns. That dismissal hurts. Real support can make all the difference.

If You're the Sexual Partner

This isn't about you, but you can be part of the solution. Changes in libido, arousal, or comfort aren't a reflection of your desirability. They're often tied to hormones, stress, pain, trauma, or medical side effects. Don't take it personally, and don't push for a quick fix. Instead, listen. Ask what they need. Support them in getting care. Not just for your relationship but also for their health and self-confidence.

- **Affirm their experience.** Believe them when they say something feels off. Even if everything *seems* fine from the outside.
- **Support without pressure.** Avoid framing care as a way to "get things back to normal." Healing is not a performance.
- **Stay engaged.** Sexuality can shift, not disappear. Be part of open, nonjudgmental conversations about what feels good, what feels off, and what support actually looks like.

If You're Coming to the Visit

But your presence can be powerful. Just by sitting in that room, you're backing their right to sexual healthcare that's real, not rushed. Let them lead, but don't be afraid to advocate if the provider starts to minimize: "This is having a real impact on their well-being, and I want to understand how we can support that together."

Scenario 15

Queer Sex Ed

Inclusive anatomy, safer sex, and reclaiming pleasure on your own terms

Maybe you already know some of this.

Maybe you're learning it for the first time.

Maybe you've pieced it together through trial and error, relying on partners to show you the ropes or Googling things you were too embarrassed to ask out loud.

However you got here, welcome.

You deserve more than scattered information and awkward conversations.

You deserve sexual health education that's actually *for you*. Not built on straight, cis, reproductive scripts that ignore how women who have sex with women actually live and love.

This is for you.

No shame. No assumptions.

Just truth, tools, and the care you've always deserved.

Bodies, Not Binaries: Real Anatomy, Real Connection

Most of us learned anatomy from outdated charts that sorted bodies into two boxes, "female" or "male," and called it a day. Real anatomy isn't that simple. Bodies are diverse. Language is personal. And what matters most is understanding how your body works and how to talk about it in ways that feel affirming and true to you.

You might use words like *vagina*, *pussy*, *clit*, *strap*, or *bits*. You might say *front hole*, *down there*, or something entirely your own. There's no right or wrong. What matters is clarity, comfort, and consent—between you and your own body, and between you and your partners.

Whether you're navigating sex with another woman for the first time or have been in queer relationships for years, one thing remains true: you deserve real sex education that honors your body, your experience, and your pleasure.

Here's what's worth knowing:

- **The clitoris is not just the small nub you can see.** It's a complex organ with internal branches that wrap around the vaginal canal. It's the primary source of pleasure for most people with this anatomy. And it's rarely taught in full.
- **Arousal and lubrication are affected by more than desire.** Hormones, stress, medications, trauma, and life stage all shape what your body does. It's normal for things to feel different over time. That's not failure, it's biology.
- **Sensation may be shaped by experience.** Trauma, dysphoria, childbirth, or surgeries can influence how you feel in your body. That doesn't make sex off-limits, it just makes communication more important.
- **Sex doesn't have to involve penetration.** Oral sex, manual stimulation, toys, body-to-body intimacy. All of it counts. You get to define what sex is, what feels good, and what feels right for you and your partner. Connection and pleasure are what matter.
- **Sex doesn't have to include orgasm.** As long as you and your partner are enjoying it, take the pressure off.
- **Language matters.** Your words for your body, and your partner's words for theirs, are part of your sexual vocabulary. Ask. Listen. Respect. That's intimacy.

You get to rewrite the script.

You don't have to mimic heteronormative models or justify what turns you on.

The Pleasure-Centered Sex Ed You Deserved

If you were taught anything about sex, it probably focused on pregnancy prevention or sexually transmitted infections (STIs) and left out queer sex entirely. When sex isn't tied to reproduction, people often assume it doesn't "count." But that couldn't be further from the truth.

When sex isn't about outcome, it can be about pleasure, creativity, healing, connection, and trust. For many women who have sex with women, that freedom opens the door to more exploration—not less.

Let's normalize:

- Sex without penetration and not seeing that as missing something
- Sex with lube, toys, fingers, mouths, bodies, and intention
- Talking about what feels good and what doesn't
- Pausing, laughing, redirecting, because sex isn't a performance
- Letting go of pressure to "do it right" or to climax

Pleasure is part of your wellness.
It's not selfish. It's not extra.
It's not reserved for straight people or for people in long-term relationships.
Pleasure is part of your sexual health, your self-knowledge, and your joy.

You Weren't Imagining It, You Were Left Out

If you have sex that falls outside straight, penis-in-vagina assumptions, chances are no one ever explained what that actually means for your health. You were likely skipped in health class, labeled "low risk," told you couldn't get STIs, that you didn't need protection, or that you only needed a gynecologist if pregnancy was the goal.

That erasure does not just create confusion. It creates harm. And much of what you were told is simply wrong.

So let's be clear:

- People having queer sex can get and pass STIs. Gender, anatomy, and the type of sex you're having matter more than labels.
- Certain infections, including bacterial vaginosis (BV), can be more common in some queer sexual networks due to shared anatomy, fluid exchange, sex toys, and gaps in affirming care, not because queer sex is "riskier."
- Queer people deserve inclusive, affirming, medically competent OB-GYN care that understands real sexual practices, not assumptions based on identity.

Bacteria, BV, and STIs: What Queer Women Deserve to Know

For way too long, sexual health has been framed around heterosexual intercourse and pregnancy prevention. That narrow lens leaves queer women underserved. Your risk doesn't disappear just because a penis isn't involved. Providers were simply never trained to talk about this. You still deserve full, informed care.

BV is more common among queer, especially when sex involves finger-to-vaginal contact, oral sex, or shared toys. BV isn't an STI, but sexual activity can disrupt the vaginal microbiome, and partners can pass that imbalance back and forth.

STIs can absolutely be transmitted without a penis involved. Oral, manual, and toy-based sex can spread infections like human papillomavirus, herpes, trichomonas, gonorrhea, chlamydia (less common, but possible), syphilis, and hepatitis. Anatomical sameness doesn't remove risks.

Barrier protection reduces microtears, friction, and bacterial or viral transmission. Routine OB-GYN care still applies: Pap tests, STI screening, and conversations about discomfort, discharge, lubrication, or pleasure are part of comprehensive care.

BV Is Real and Often Recurring

If you've ever dealt with persistent discharge, a "fishy" odor, irritation, or pelvic heaviness, it may have been BV, even if no one ever named it. BV is common, underdiscussed, particularly in people having queer sex..

What increases risk among WSW:

- Sex without barriers (oral, fingers, shared toys)
- Sharing toys without cleaning or using condoms between partners
- New or multiple partners
- Stress or hormonal shifts
- Douching or scented products
- A history of BV

What to do:

- Ask for a vaginal swab so you're not guessing.
- Treat with oral or vaginal antibiotics if needed. Have your partner be treated as well.
- Avoid scented soaps or douching, they destabilize vaginal flora.
- Consider probiotics, pH-balancing gels, or over-the-counter boric acid to support recovery.

What Queer Safe Sex Looks Like

Let's redefine what protection means.

Barriers + Practices That Matter

- Condoms on shared toys
- Gloves for manual sex (especially with long nails or small cuts)
- Dental dams or cut condoms for oral sex
- Lube to reduce friction and prevent microtears
- Toy cleaner after every use to reduce risk of infections or pH imbalance

Pleasure, Not Just Prevention

Too often queer sex gets framed around risk, or ignored entirely. But pleasure matters, too. Many individuals may never hear that arousal, lubrication, exploration, and enjoyment all deserve space.

Let's shift the focus:

- It's okay if arousal takes time.
- Lube is your friend, especially with hormonal changes or menopause.
- Sex can be playful, emotional, creative, not just penetrative.
- Toys, positions, pace, and pressure should match what feels good to you.
- There is no "right" way to have sex.

You are allowed to explore.
You are allowed to set boundaries.
You are allowed to center pleasure.

Communication Builds Safety and Trust

Queer sex doesn't have a universal script. Every partner brings different experiences, histories, bodies, and boundaries to the table.

You don't need to guess. Try asking:

- "What feels good to you?"
- "Is there anything you'd rather avoid?"
- "Do you want to use protection tonight?"

- "Is it okay if I check in during?"
- "Do you want to try something new or stick to what feels good?"

Workbook: Claiming Care, Pleasure, and Safety on Your Terms

I want to ...

☐ Learn more about queer sexual health that reflects my reality
☐ Talk to my partner(s) about protection, pleasure, and communication
☐ Understand BV, STIs, and vaginal health in queer relationships
☐ Find a provider who respects my identity and offers inclusive care
☐ Reclaim the language, practices, and definitions that feel right for me
☐ Let go of shame and explore sex on my own terms

Questions I have about my body, health, or pleasure:

_____

_____

_____

Support I want or need from a partner:

_____

_____

_____

What I want sex and intimacy to feel like:

_____

_____

_____

Support I want or need from my clinician:

_____

_____

_____

Reminders to come back to:

- My sex life doesn't need to look like anyone else's to be real.
- I'm allowed to ask questions. Even if I think I "should" know already.
- I deserve healthcare that sees the whole me, not just the parts that fit a checkbox.
- Pleasure isn't extra. It's part of my wellness.
- There is no one right way to be queer, to have sex, or to be in my body.

For Support People

They may have gone years without being taught how their body works or how to navigate queer sex safely. They might still be unlearning shame, myths, or outdated scripts about what counts as sex—or who deserves pleasure.

Be affirming, not assuming. Don't assume past experience means confidence or that curiosity means inexperience. Let them lead the conversation about what feels good, what language they use for their body, and what they need from you.

Be part of their safety. Offer to clean toys together. Use gloves or barriers without making it awkward. Normalize checking in before, during, and after, especially if trauma or dysphoria is part of their story.

Reinforce what's real. Queer sex is real sex. Queer pleasure is real pleasure. They deserve partners who treat their body with care, respect, and joy, not as an exception to some made-up rulebook.

Scenario 16

Family Expansion Conversations That Don't Assume

Whether you want kids, don't want kids, or aren't sure, how to take control of the narrative

Fertility Isn't Just a Given. It's a Choice

Fertility care shouldn't come with assumptions. But far too often, it does.

Providers assume you want kids. That you want them now. That your biological clock is ticking and your priorities should be, too. And if you *don't* want kids? You're told you'll change your mind. That you're too young to know. That permanent options aren't "appropriate."

Let's be clear: fertility is personal. It doesn't follow a script. And no matter where you stand—whether you want kids someday, never, or don't know yet, you deserve care that reflects *your* values, *your* timeline, and *your* autonomy.

There are four scenarios we'll explore in this chapter. All of them are valid.

I: I'm not ready now, but I know that I want kids someday. This scenario is about curiosity and preparation. Maybe you're in your 20s or early 30s and thinking ahead, or maybe you're 38 and starting to worry about time. You want to understand what your body is doing now, and what your options are if you want to preserve fertility for later. We'll help you prep to ask the right questions. About testing, egg freezing, and timelines.

II: I don't want kids now, but I'd like to leave the door open. This one is for the "maybe later" crowd. You might be interested in preserving fertility while you figure things out, or just want to keep future options on the table. We'll walk through how to approach this with your provider without feeling pressured into a decision you're not ready to make.

III: I don't want children, now or ever. You're clear on your choice, and you're tired of having to defend it every single year when you see your OB-GYN. You deserve care that respects your autonomy without caveats, lectures, or "what if you regret it" warnings. We'll give you scripts for shutting down the yearly fertility assumption and asking for permanent birth control if that's your choice.

IV: I want to have a baby now, and I don't have a partner. You're ready for parenthood, and you're planning on doing it solo. This often referred to as single mother by choice or SMBC. Maybe you're exploring donor insemination or just wondering what this path might look like. We'll help you prep questions and navigate conversations that center your agency and your plan.

Fertility planning deserves time, not an afterthought at the end of your annual. These conversations, whether about preserving, pursuing, or opting out, deserve space to breathe. If you want to explore your options in depth, schedule a dedicated fertility or family planning consult. That's where you'll actually have time to discuss testing, timelines, procedures, and next steps without being rushed or redirected.

And if you're done with the conversation? That's worth saying. too: "Please note in my chart that I do not want children. If that ever changes, I'll bring it up."

Pre-Visit Planning

I: I'm Not Ready Now, but I Know That I Want Kids Someday

You want to be a parent in the future, but the timing isn't right for now. You're trying to balance your health, your goals, your finances, and your life. You're not looking for pressure, you're looking for a plan. This stage isn't about rushing into decisions; it's about learning what's possible, understanding your body, and hearing clear, honest answers so you can decide what feels right for *you*. You deserve information and guidance, not fear, guilt, or panic. The goal is to walk away with clarity and confidence so you feel empowered in your timeline and in your choices.

What to ask:

- What age-related changes should I be aware of in terms of fertility?
- What testing can help me understand my current fertility status?
- Are there ways to track my cycle or ovulation over time to spot changes early?
- Is there value in doing baseline fertility testing like Anti-Müllerian hormone or antral follicle count?
- How reliable are fertility tests in predicting my personal chances of conceiving later?
- How often should fertility testing be repeated if I'm not trying to conceive yet?
- What is egg freezing and when should I consider it?
- What does the whole process entail? Cost, meds, procedures, follow-up?
- What other fertility preservation options should I know about?

What to prepare:

- What is your general timeline (roughly)?
- Do you have any known risks or conditions that might affect fertility?
- Does your insurance cover egg freezing or fertility benefits?

II: I Don't Want Kids Now, but I'd Like to Leave the Door Open

You're in the "not now, maybe later" zone. You're not closing the door, you just don't need it wide open either. You're exploring fertility as a *possibility*, not a promise. You might want the option someday, or you might not. And that's okay. This stage is about curiosity, not commitment. You deserve space to ask questions, understand your body, and weigh your options without being rushed or judged. Maybe building a family doesn't have to mean biological children for you. Or maybe you just want to leave every door unlocked until you're ready to choose. What matters is having good information and guidance, not pressure or panic.

In addition to the questions from the preceding section, you can also consider asking the following:

- How can I preserve optionality without feeling pressured? What's a realistic timeline for deciding?
- What costs should I plan for in the future if I pursue preservation?
- If I choose not to freeze eggs right now, what else can I do to monitor fertility over the next few years?

What to prepare:

- Do you want to make decisions now or just gather information?
- Are you looking for peace of mind or an actual next step?
- What kind of information helps you feel grounded instead of panicked?
- If you decide you do want kids later on, are you open to non-biological children?

III: I Don't Want Kids, Now or Ever

You've made a clear and thoughtful decision. You don't want children, now or ever. You're not looking for validation, just respectful, competent care that aligns with your choice. You don't need to defend your decision or explain it away; you simply deserve providers who take you at your word, document your preferences, and offer options that match your goals. And importantly, you don't want to have to say it every single year over and over again at your visits.

What to ask:

- Can we document my decision clearly in the chart?
- What are my options for longer acting or permanent contraception?
- Are you comfortable offering sterilization procedures to people without children?
- If you won't perform sterilization on someone without children, can you refer me to someone who is?

What to know about permanent sterilization:

If you're interested in a permanent method, it's worth knowing that a tubal ligation (having your "tubes tied") isn't the most common approach anymore. Today, many clinicians perform a bilateral salpingectomy, which removes the fallopian tubes entirely. It's permanent, highly effective, and may also reduce the risk of ovarian cancers.

If you're in a committed partnership and have reached a shared decision not to have children, a vasectomy can be a great option to discuss. Vasectomies are a simple outpatient procedure that cuts or blocks the vas deferens (the tubes that carry sperm), takes about 15–30 minutes, and has a much shorter recovery period. It's worth having an open, honest conversation with your provider, and with each other. about which route feels best for your bodies, your values, and your long-term goals.

IV: I Want a Baby Now, and I Don't Have a Partner

You're ready to become a parent, even if you're doing it solo. You may be considering IUI, donor sperm, or just want to talk about your options. You deserve care that supports your decision and your timeline.

This path takes planning, clarity, and emotional readiness, but it also takes information. A good clinician should help you understand your fertility baseline, walk you through medical options, and connect you with trusted fertility specialists, counselors, and donor resources. It's okay to feel both certain and overwhelmed; those two things can coexist. The goal here isn't to have every answer, it's to build a road map that makes the process feel possible and supported.

Be up front with your clinician: "I'm planning to pursue parenthood on my own and want to understand what my next steps should be." You're not asking for permission. You're setting the tone for the care you deserve: informed, respectful, and rooted in the belief that solo parenthood is not a last resort, but a valid, empowered choice.

What to ask:

- What fertility testing should we start with (e.g., AMH, follicle-stimulating hormone, ultrasound)?
- Can you manage any of this process here, or will you refer me to a reproductive endocrinologist or fertility clinic?
- What are the differences among IUI, in vitro fertilization, and home insemination in terms of success rates, cost, and logistics?
- Can you walk me through how donor sperm works? How do I choose, store, and use it safely?
- What are the emotional and legal considerations I should plan for when using donor sperm?

What to prepare:

- What's your general timeline or readiness? Are you hoping to try soon or gathering information first?
- Do you already have a fertility clinic or would you like referrals?
- Have you researched potential donor options, sperm banks, or known donor agreements?
- What kind of emotional and practical support system do you have in place (friends, family, community)?
- Do you want to explore financial planning or grants for fertility treatment?

For Support People

They're navigating deeply personal decisions about family planning while also fielding societal pressure about what they *should* want. What they need most from you is support for their actual desires, not your assumptions and not the world's expectations.

Support their timeline. Don't pressure them toward any particular decision about children or fertility. Their feelings may evolve, and that's completely okay.

Respect uncertainty. If they're unsure about wanting children, be a steady presence as they explore what's right for them. Support doesn't mean pushing for a resolution, it means giving space to figure it out.

Help understand options, not steer them. If they want to explore egg freezing or permanent contraception, walk alongside them. Not ahead of them. Help with research if they ask, but leave the final say to them.

Navigating dual roles. If you're their partner, you're likely balancing two roles: supporting their decisions *and* processing your own feelings. You might feel disappointed, relieved, confused, or conflicted about what's being discussed. That's normal. The challenge is holding space for your emotions *without* letting them override their autonomy.

When your feelings conflict. If their decisions around fertility bring up strong emotions for you, it's okay to feel what you feel. Just separate your emotional processing from the clinical visit. There's room for both of your needs in the relationship. However, in the exam room, your role is to support their choices, not shift the focus to your own.

If you're joining the visit. Keep the spotlight on their goals. Whether they want to talk about permanent contraception, fertility preservation, or nothing at all, follow their lead. You can always have deeper conversations later. In the moment, be their advocate.

Scenario 17

Aging and Egg Freezing: What You Should Know

Not sure whether to freeze your eggs, track your cycle, or ignore the noise?

Before You Walk In

You're in your late 20s, 30s, or early 40s and suddenly everyone has an opinion about your biological clock. Your mom asks when you're giving her grandchildren. Your friends are either frantically freezing eggs or posting pregnancy announcements. Articles scream about "fertility cliffs" at 35, while Instagram ads promise egg freezing will solve everything. Yet you also see celebrities having kids at 45 and wonder if it's all overblown.

You're trying to figure things out: *What's actually true? What are my real options? And how do I make informed decisions about my fertility without either panicking or pretending age doesn't matter?*

This scenario isn't about telling you what to do with your reproductive timeline. It's about helping you understand what's happening in your body as you age, what options exist to preserve fertility, and how to navigate the healthcare system to get the information and care you need. Whether that's fertility testing, an egg-freezing consult, or just a conversation that leaves you feeling more grounded.

Understanding Fertility and Age: The Real Story

Let's start with what's actually true about fertility and aging. Most of what we've been told is either fear-based ("your clock is ticking!") or falsely reassuring ("you can wait as long as you want"). The truth lives somewhere in between.

You're born with all the eggs you'll ever have, around one to two million. By puberty, that number drops to about 400,000. Each month, roughly 1,000 eggs are lost, whether or not you ovulate, and whether or not you've been on birth control. In your 30s, the rate of loss accelerates, and both the *quantity* and *quality* of eggs begin to decline. That's why miscarriage rates and chromosomal abnormalities rise with age.

Being on birth control doesn't "save" or "use up" eggs, it simply pauses ovulation. When you stop, your fertility reflects your age, not how long you were on the pill.

Let's talk about that "fertility cliff" at 35. It's not a cliff, it's a slope. Fertility starts to decline in your early 30s, more noticeably after 35, but many people still conceive naturally in their late 30s and early 40s. It just becomes less predictable and can take longer.

In practice:

Everyone's fertility journey looks different. Age is a factor, but not the only one. Conditions like polycystic ovary syndrome or endometriosis, lifestyle, and genetics all play a role. The key is understanding *your* body, not just statistics. If you're not ready for kids now, egg freezing can extend your options. If you're unsure whether you want them at all, that's okay, too. The goal is not panic, but perspective.

What About the Term *Advanced Maternal Age*?

Yes, it sounds outdated, and it can feel patronizing, but in medicine, *advanced maternal age (AMA)* isn't an insult. It's a clinical term used to guide care and coverage for patients over 35.

Here's what it really means:

- **It's tied to data.** Risk for miscarriage, chromosomal changes, and pregnancy complications increases with age.
- **It can help with insurance.** Many plans require the AMA label to cover extra screening or genetic testing.
- **It signals closer monitoring.** Providers use it to justify additional care and testing, it's not judgment.

Starting the Conversation and Getting Referred

Your OB-GYN can help you start exploring fertility preservation, but they're not the ones who manage egg freezing or advanced treatment. Think of them as your launch point—the person who orders initial tests and connects you with the right specialists.

What your gynecologist can do:

- Explain fertility basics and how hormones change with age.
- Order initial labs for anti-Müllerian hormone, follicle-stimulating hormone, and thyroid-stimulating hormone to check ovarian reserve.
- Discuss timelines and next steps.
- Refer you to a reproductive endocrinologist.

What requires a fertility specialist:

- Comprehensive fertility evaluation and treatment plan
- Egg freezing consultation and retrieval procedure
- Ovarian stimulation and monitoring
- Success rate, cost, and timeline counseling

Understanding Egg Freezing

Egg freezing typically involves a short but intense process. Over about 8 to 14 days, you'll give yourself daily hormonal injections to encourage multiple eggs to mature at once. During that time, you'll have frequent ultrasounds and blood draws so your care team can track your progress and adjust medications as needed. When the follicles are ready, a brief outpatient procedure is done under light sedation to retrieve the eggs. You'll be asleep but breathing on your own, and the procedure usually takes less than 30 minutes. The mature eggs are then frozen and stored for potential future use.

Physically, most people experience temporary bloating, cramping, or breast tenderness from the hormonal stimulation. You'll likely need a day of rest after the retrieval itself, but recovery is generally quick. Emotionally, though, the process can take more out of you than you might expect. Hormone shifts can make you feel weepy or irritable, and the frequent appointments can leave you feeling both accomplished and completely wiped out. It's common to feel proud and empowered one moment, then uncertain or vulnerable the next.

Give yourself space to recover, both physically and mentally. Plan for rest, eat well, hydrate, and if you can, line up a calm evening or a friend who makes you feel steady. Egg freezing can be an empowering choice, but it's also a demanding one. Allow yourself the grace to rest, process, and acknowledge what a big step it is to take ownership of your reproductive future.

Understanding Insurance Coverage and What It Might Cost

Coverage for fertility care and egg freezing varies wildly depending on where you live, whom you work for, and what kind of insurance you have. There's no national standard, just a patchwork of state laws, employer perks, and insurance fine print that can make an already emotional decision feel even more confusing.

Here's the reality:

- Only about half of US states have any fertility coverage mandates, and most apply only to employer-based insurance, not individual or federal plans.
- Even when fertility coverage exists, it usually applies to *infertility treatment* (meaning you must prove you've been trying to conceive for a year), not elective or "social" egg freezing.
- Coverage is more likely if your fertility is at risk due to medical reasons like chemotherapy, endometriosis, or ovarian surgery.
- Some employers, especially in tech, law, and finance, offer egg freezing as part of their benefits. These plans may include one or two cycles, partial medication coverage, and a few years of storage, but they're the exception, not the rule.
- Medications, anesthesia, and long-term storage are often billed separately. And those costs add up fast.

Typical out-of-pocket costs (US averages):

- $10,000–$20,000 per egg freezing cycle (does not include meds)
- $3,000–$6,000 for fertility medications per cycle
- $500–$1,500 per year for egg storage
- $5,000–$10,000 for thawing, fertilization, and transfer later

Many people need more than one retrieval cycle to reach their goal number of eggs so total costs can easily climb into the $20,000–$40,000+ range.

Questions to ask your insurance or human resources representative:

- Does my plan cover fertility preservation or egg freezing? And under what conditions?
- Is there a difference between "medical" and "elective" coverage?
- Are medications, anesthesia, and annual storage included or billed separately?
- Do I need prior authorization or a referral before I start?
- Which clinics or specialists are in-network?
- Are there annual or lifetime maximums for fertility benefits?

If your state doesn't have a fertility mandate, or your insurance excludes elective freezing, ask clinics about cash-pay discounts, financing, or grants. Some fertility centers offer payment plans or refund programs based on outcomes.

And if you live in a state like New York, Illinois, Massachusetts, or Colorado, you may have stronger protections that cover fertility preservation for both medical and nonmedical reasons. Always confirm coverage in writing before starting any cycle.

Making the Decision: Is Egg Freezing Right for You?

It might make sense if the following is true:

- You're not ready for kids but know you want them someday.
- You're single and want to preserve options.
- You're facing a medical treatment that could affect fertility.

It might not be necessary if the following is true:

- You're planning to try soon.
- You're unsure whether you want kids.
- You're open to donor eggs or adoption later.
- It would cause financial strain.

Pre-Visit Planning: Based on Your Scenario

Your visit might focus on education, testing, or referral. It's okay to ask for time to explore options without committing to anything.

What's prompting this conversation?

- ☐ I'm feeling pressure.
- ☐ I want kids someday but not for several years.
- ☐ I'm single and want to preserve options.
- ☐ My partner and I aren't ready but are worried about waiting.
- ☐ I've heard about egg freezing and want to understand it.
- ☐ I want to know my fertility status before deciding.
- ☐ Other: _____

Questions for Your Fertility Specialist

About the process:

- How many eggs would you expect to retrieve at my age?
- What are the risks and side effects?
- How many cycles might I need?

About timing:

- Is this the best time for me to freeze?
- What happens if I wait a year or two?
- How long can eggs stay frozen?

About costs:

- What's the full cost including medications and storage?
- Does insurance cover any part of it?
- Are there payment plans or grants?

About the future:

- What are my chances of pregnancy using frozen eggs?
- How does this differ from in vitro fertilization?
- What would my next steps be if I decide to use them later?

Questions for Your Future Timeline

If you want kids someday but not now:

- What's my ideal timeline?
- How can I prepare emotionally and financially?
- What's my backup plan if conception doesn't come easily?

If you're undecided about kids:

- How important is having biological children?
- Would egg freezing help me feel calmer—or more pressured?
- What would I regret more: doing it or not doing it?
- Am I doing this for myself—or because I think I "should"?

For Support People

They're navigating an emotional, physical, and often expensive decision all while facing outside pressure and internal uncertainty. They may feel overwhelmed by timelines, test results, or expectations about what they "should" do. Your job isn't to solve it. It's to stay grounded with them in the unknown.

Support looks like the following:

- Asking, "Do you want to talk through options or just vent today?"
- Holding space for indecision without rushing a conclusion.
- Going with them to appointments or offering to help with research.
- Reminding them they have time, autonomy, and support no matter what they choose.
- Avoiding comments about "when" they'll have kids. Stay focused on if, when, and how they want to.

The best thing you can do? Trust them to lead the conversation, and follow with compassion—not an agenda.

Scenario 18

It's Time to Try: Getting Pregnant on Purpose

Ready to start trying to get pregnant or perhaps you just pulled the goalie, let's work on understanding your body, your options, and your next steps

This is the space where excitement meets uncertainty. Even for people who've spent years trying *not* to get pregnant, the shift to trying *on purpose* can feel surprisingly unfamiliar. You might assume it's as simple as stopping birth control and waiting, but soon find yourself deep in articles about ovulation timing, sperm health, prenatals, and fertility myths. It's easy to feel both curious and overwhelmed.

This scenario isn't about fertility treatment or diagnosing infertility, it's about building a foundation. Understanding what's happening in your body, how conception really works, and what steps actually matter can make this process feel more grounded and less like a guessing game. Whether you're hoping for pregnancy soon or simply want to begin thoughtfully, this guide walks you through how to prepare your body, understand your cycle, and recognize when it might be time to ask for support.

Before You Begin: Setting Expectations

Trying to conceive is one of those experiences that's both deeply personal and completely universal, and yet no one really prepares you for how variable it can be. For most couples with regular cycles and no known conditions, conception can take several months. In fact, it's entirely normal for it to take up to a year, even when everything is working exactly as it should. That doesn't mean something is wrong; it means human reproduction is complex and not always efficient.

Cycles can vary, timing can be tricky, and stress, sleep, travel, or illness can all affect ovulation. So while tracking your cycle and timing intercourse can be helpful, it's also important to protect your mental health along the way. Trying to conceive can easily shift from exciting to all-consuming. And that's when it helps to zoom out and remember: this is a process, not a test of your body or your worth.

Go into it informed, not anxious. Know what's within your control, like nutrition, timing, and lifestyle factors, and what's simply part of biology doing its unpredictable thing. Understanding that range of "normal" can make all the difference between feeling discouraged and feeling grounded.

Understanding Ovulation, Timing, and Tracking

When it comes to conception, timing really is everything. Most people aren't taught much about their cycle and knowing when you actually *can* conceive is one of the most empowering things you can learn about your body.

The Fertile Window: When Pregnancy Can Happen

You can get pregnant only during a short window each cycle: the five days before ovulation and the day of ovulation itself.

- **Sperm** can live in the reproductive tract for up to five days.
- **The egg** survives for only about 12–24 hours after ovulation.
  That means sex in the few days *before* ovulation gives sperm time to be waiting in the right place when the egg is released.

A common mistake is counting forward from your period. Ovulation does not happen 14 days after your period starts. It usually happens about 14 days before your next period. So if your cycle is 30 days long, ovulation is more likely around day 16, not day 14.

Timed Intercourse Basics

Cycle day 1 is the first day of your period. If you're trying to conceive, timing matters. For people with a 28- to 30-day cycle, the fertile window typically between cycle days 10 and 18.

Having sex every one to two days during this window gives you the best chance of pregnancy. Having sex more often than that does not improve outcomes and can reduce sperm count, which is why frequency matters as much as timing.

If you're using ovulation predictor kits (OPKs), a positive result means ovulation is likely to occur within the next 24–48 hours. This is one of the most important times to have sex if pregnancy is the goal.

How to Track Your Cycle (Without Losing Your Mind)

You don't need to track every variable or buy every gadget. The goal is simply to notice patterns and confirm when ovulation is happening.

- **Period-tracking apps.** Helpful for spotting trends over time
- **OPKs.** Urine tests that detect the luteinizing hormone surge that triggers ovulation, this is helpful to know when you've got the best chance
- **Cervical mucus changes.** Looking for clear, stretchy, slippery discharge; that's your body's natural fertility signal
- **Basal body temperature.** Your resting temperature rising slightly after ovulation, confirming ovulation has happened but can't predict it ahead of time
- **Calendar method.** Estimating ovulation based on average cycle length can be fine when you're just getting started, but it's the least precise.

When Do You Need a Visit?

You don't have to see a provider the moment you decide to start trying. Plenty of people begin by learning their cycles, starting prenatals, and seeing what happens. But if you're unsure what's normal, want reassurance, or are managing health factors, it's completely fine (and often helpful) to get support early.

You might consider scheduling a preconception or fertility visit if any of the following are true:

- You're not sure which supplements or vitamins to start.
- You're coming off birth control and have questions about what to expect.
- You'd like help learning how to track ovulation.
- You want to review your medications or health conditions before pregnancy.
- You're interested in preconception bloodwork or genetic carrier screening.
- Your cycles are irregular or missing altogether.
- You've had a miscarriage and want support trying again.

You don't need to have everything figured out before reaching out. Curiosity is enough reason to make an appointment. A good clinician will meet you where you are, with information, not pressure.

Prenatal Preparation: What to Do Before Pregnancy

Whether you're months away from trying or just pulled the goalie, there are a few easy steps that make a real difference before conception.

- **Start a prenatal vitamin** ideally two to three months before trying.
- **Check your rubella immunity** (via IgG titer). If you're not immune, get vaccinated and wait one month before conceiving.
- **Consider genetic carrier screening,** especially if you have Jewish, Mediterranean, Black, or Southeast Asian ancestry, or a family history of inherited conditions.
- **Review medications and supplements.** Some aren't safe in early pregnancy. Talk to your prescribers about your plans so they can adjust ahead of time.
- **No need to wait after stopping birth control.** You can conceive as soon as ovulation resumes, though cycles may take one to three months to find their new rhythm.
- **Know when to test.** If your period is late, take a pregnancy test. Don't assume your cycle's "off." Post-pill symptoms and early pregnancy can feel similar, and a test gives clarity.

When It's Time for a Fertility Evaluation

If you've been trying and not getting pregnant, here's when it makes sense to check in:

- **Under 35:** after **12 months** of regular, unprotected sex without conception
- **35 or older:** after **6 months**

That doesn't mean waiting in silence until those marks hit, those are just benchmarks for when a full fertility workup is recommended. You should check in sooner if any of the following are true:

- Your cycles are irregular, extremely short, or very long.
- You've been diagnosed with polycystic ovary syndrome, endometriosis, or thyroid disorders.

- You've had pelvic surgery or infections that could affect fertility.
- You or your partner have known reproductive health concerns.

Getting a fertility consult isn't a failure, it's a chance to understand your body more deeply. The goal isn't rushing to treatment; it's gaining clarity so you can make informed choices about next steps.

What About My Partner's Fertility?

Male factor infertility contributes to nearly half of all fertility challenges. Even though one partner carries the pregnancy, both bodies matter. and it's worth remembering that conception is a team process.

A semen analysis is a quick, noninvasive test that checks sperm count, movement (motility), and shape (morphology). It's one of the simplest and least expensive fertility tests available, and it can offer helpful clarity early on.

That said, you don't need to rush into testing right away. Most couples start by learning cycles, timing sex during the fertile window, and giving it a few months before pursuing evaluation. If you're curious—or if there are known health factors like prior injuries, surgeries, or hormone issues—it's easy to request a test sooner.

Ask your provider these questions:

- "When would it make sense for my partner to get a semen analysis?"
- "Can we order one proactively, or should we wait a few cycles first?"

Starting with both partners in mind keeps the focus balanced. Fertility isn't a solo story, it's a shared one, and information on both sides can make the path forward feel clearer and less stressful.

Emotions in the Trying Stage

Trying to get pregnant is often framed as a time of joy and excitement, but for many people, it feels more like a mix of hope, fear, and uncertainty. That's normal. You can feel grateful and terrified, ready and hesitant, all at once.

You might also realize there's never a "perfect time." Careers, finances, relationships, something will always feel unfinished. Most people start trying when it feels *good enough*, not perfectly aligned.

No one talks enough about how *scary* it can be to start trying. You might feel pressure to be excited, but instead feel anxious about what's next. What if it takes a while? What if something goes wrong? What if life doesn't look the way you expected? Those feelings don't mean you're ungrateful or not ready; they mean you're human.

And then there's the part no one really warns you about: the logistics of it all. When sex becomes something to schedule and optimize, it can feel like work. It's no longer fun, spontaneous, or sexy. That's okay, too. It doesn't mean your relationship is broken or that something's wrong with you.

Give yourself permission to hold all of it. The joy, the worry, the doubt, the occasional frustration that "baby-making sex" feels more clinical than passionate. None of it disqualifies you from this experience. It's all part of the process: messy, emotional, and completely human.

Supporting Each Other While Trying

If you're doing this with a partner, remember that you're both navigating uncertainty, just in different ways. The best thing you can do is communicate early and often. About hopes, fears, sex, and the emotional toll of the waiting game.

- **Talk about expectations** before you start testing or timing. How much do you want to track? How often do you want to have sex? How will you handle stress or disappointment?
- **Share how you each cope.** Some people want to talk constantly, others prefer distraction. Neither is wrong but it helps to name the difference.
- **Protect intimacy.** Trying to conceive can quickly make sex feel like a chore. Build in connection that's not about ovulation: walks, laughter, affection.
- **Stay on the same team.** When conception takes longer than expected, it's easy to start blaming yourself or each other. Remember: fertility is shared biology, not personal failure.

However this chapter feels, whether you're excited, unsure, impatient, or scared, you're not alone. It's messy, it's emotional, and it's deeply human.

For Support People

They're stepping into a new chapter. Sometimes with excitement, sometimes with quiet anxiety. Trying to conceive can feel like a mix of anticipation, pressure, and unpredictability. Your role is to be steady support, not another source of stress.

Supporting emotional balance. Ask what kind of support they need. Some want shared tracking and planning, others need space and reassurance. Don't assume, ask.

Being present, not pressuring. This process isn't just about outcomes. Stay connected to the journey, not just the pregnancy test. Avoid pushing timelines or milestones that might not match their reality.

Sharing the work. If you're the partner, take on your share of the research, logistics, and emotional labor. If you're a friend, offer to help them find info, attend visits, or just be there on hard days.

Honoring their pace. Not everyone wants to talk about it all the time. Check in without hovering. Support breaks in tracking or trying without judgment.

If you're joining for a visit. Help them advocate for clear information and supportive care. Make sure the provider includes both of you (if applicable), but always follow their lead. Your job is to center their experience, not your own expectations.

Scenario 19

Starting Infertility Conversations

When trying isn't working, here's how to ask for answers, get support, and advocate for care that doesn't treat you like a number

Trying to get pregnant and not having it happen can feel like being trapped in an endless waiting room, month after month of hope, disappointment, and "maybe next time." You're charting cycles, tracking ovulation, taking your vitamins, doing everything "right" and still, nothing. It's not just physically draining; it's emotionally exhausting.

Wherever you are in this process know that you are not alone. You may feel confused, frustrated, hopeful, heartbroken, or all of the above.

Clinically, infertility is defined as *12 months of unprotected sex without pregnancy if you're under 35, or 6 months if you're over 35*. But those timelines are guidelines, not rules. If your periods are irregular, if you've had prior pelvic surgeries or infections, if your partner has a known fertility concern, or if you just know in your gut that something's off, it's okay to speak up sooner.

This next section walks you through what those next steps look like: when to seek additional workup, what tests to expect, and how to advocate for care that meets you with information and empathy, not dismissal.

What An Initial Fertility Workup Might Include

For you (the partner with a uterus):

- Hormone labs (anti-Müllerian hormone, follicle-stimulating hormone, luteinizing hormone, estradiol, thyroid-stimulating hormone, prolactin) often drawn on cycle day 3
- Transvaginal ultrasound to assess follicle count and uterine lining
- Hysterosalpingogram to check fallopian tube patency

For Your Male Partner: Don't Skip the Sperm Check

If you're planning a pregnancy with a partner who produces sperm, a semen analysis is a key part of the fertility puzzle.

A semen analysis looks at the following information:

- **Sperm count**—how many sperm are present
- **Motility**—how well the sperm swim
- **Morphology**—the shape and structure of the sperm

Here's why it matters:

About 30–40% of infertility cases are caused by male-factor issues alone, and in another 20% or so, sperm health contributes alongside other factors. That means sperm-related issues are involved in roughly half of all infertility cases, yet they're often one of the last things anyone checks.

Too often, the focus is placed entirely on the person with ovaries, as if it's their sole responsibility to figure out what's wrong, freeze their eggs, or "try harder." But if you're trying to conceive as a couple, you deserve a full picture of what's going on. Don't let the burden fall on one person just because that's what the system traditionally does.

Semen analysis is noninvasive and relatively low cost. It can be a powerful step in making informed choices, especially if you're freezing eggs, trying to conceive soon, or facing challenges getting pregnant.

What to Know About Insurance

Fertility care coverage varies widely depending on your insurance plan and state you're insured. Unfortunately, many plans offer limited or no coverage at all for advanced fertility treatments. However, certain testing and basic workup steps are often covered under general gynecologic care or diagnostic codes. That's why it may be helpful to begin with your OB-GYN if they do this before jumping straight to a fertility specialist.

Ask these questions:

- "Which parts of this evaluation are covered by insurance?"
- "Are there specific billing codes we can use to improve the chances of coverage?"
- "If I'm referred to a reproductive endocrinologist, how does that change what's covered or not?"
- "Do I need prior authorization before starting any tests or treatments?"

Always call your insurance provider or check your plan documents to confirm the following:

- What fertility-related services are covered and if it varies based on where it's performed
- Whether any fertility medications or labs are included and if it varies based on where it's prescribed or drawn
- If a referral is required
- What your out-of-pocket responsibilities are

Understanding the financial side early can help you avoid surprises and may influence whether it makes sense to stay within your general OB-GYN's care, find a new OB-GYN, or move to a reproductive endocrinologist (REI) sooner.

The Fertility Runway

No matter where you are in this process, you deserve care that meets you with clarity, compassion, and respect, and a path forward that feels informed, not intimidating.

I often explain fertility care as a runway. There are multiple stages, each designed to help you move forward one step at a time. You may not need to leap straight into the most invasive or expensive options if that doesn't feel comfortable.

Here's what the runway can look like:

- **Cycle support and timed intercourse.** Using ovulation tracking, medications, or lifestyle adjustments to improve timing and optimize natural conception.
- **Oral medication cycles.** Medications like Clomid or Letrozole can help regulate or stimulate ovulation. These are often first-line treatments prescribed by an OB-GYN and may be combined with monitoring to time intercourse.

- **Intrauterine insemination (IUI).** A more targeted next step, where sperm are placed directly into the uterus near ovulation to increase the chances of fertilization. This is often combined with oral medication cycles.
- **IVF.** A more advanced option involving injectable hormones to stimulate multiple eggs, retrieval in a clinic setting, and fertilization in a lab before transferring embryos back into the uterus.

Each step has its place, and each comes with its own benefits, costs, and emotional weight. The key is finding the balance. It's important to move forward without rushing, but also recognize that time matters, especially as age and egg quality play a role.

Waiting too long can limit options, but moving too quickly can lead to unnecessary stress, cost, or intervention.

This guide focuses on what most general OB-GYNs can do: the initial workup, basic labs, and first-line medication cycles. If your OB-GYN doesn't offer any fertility management you can consider seeing another OB-GYN who may or going to REI right away. And if you've already done these and still aren't pregnant, that's when it's time to see a REI for advanced testing or treatments like IUI or IVF which is beyond the scope of what we'll cover here.

The Emotional Side of the Waiting

Infertility isn't just a medical diagnosis. It's an emotional marathon.

You start out hopeful, then the waiting begins. Each month brings a new wave of planning, testing, waiting, and ultimately disappointment. You might feel like your body is failing you, or that you're the only one still waiting while everyone else moves forward. It can start to impact your sense of time, your relationships, even your self-worth. You are not alone if you feel this way and if any of that sounds familiar, please know this: *nothing about this is your fault.*

It's okay if you need to step back from conversations that feel triggering, or from the constant hum of pregnancy announcements on social media. It's okay if you want to grieve what you thought this would look like. It's okay to not want to go to baby showers. And it's also okay to find joy in other parts of your life while still wanting this deeply.

Support matters here. That could mean therapy, a fertility support group, or just one friend who lets you talk without trying to fix it. You deserve space to process all of this, not just the science of fertility, but the experience of it, too.

Because trying shouldn't mean suffering in silence. You deserve compassion, connection, and care at every stage of the journey.

What to Say to Your Provider

Starting this conversation can feel vulnerable. Maybe you're scared of saying it out loud or scared of the next steps. There's no "perfect" way to start this conversation, just the one that gets you closer to being heard. The goal isn't to sound polished or prepared. It's to show up as you are, with your questions, your fears, and your right to real answers.

Here are a few ways to start:

- **If you're not sure where to begin.** "We've been trying for a while, and I'm starting to worry something might be off. Can we talk about what testing or next steps make sense?"
- **If you want to be proactive.** "I know I'm under 35, but I don't want to wait a full year before we look into this. Can we start with some initial workup?"
- **If you're overwhelmed by the options.** Can you walk me through all the options, what usually comes first, reasons to start where, and what makes sense in my situation?"
- **If you need emotional space acknowledged.** "This process has been harder than I expected. I'd appreciate if we could talk about both the medical next steps and how to manage the stress around it."

For Support People

Infertility affects relationships and friendships, but the medical and social burden often falls disproportionately on the person with the uterus. Whether you're their partner or close friend, they need you to help share the emotional load rather than letting them carry this alone.

Sharing the emotional load. If you're the partner, this isn't just "her problem." Both of you need support and both should be involved in testing and treatment decisions. If you're a friend, understand that infertility can consume someone's emotional bandwidth and adjust your expectations accordingly.

(continued)

(continued)

Managing relationship stress. Infertility can strain partnerships and friendships. Partners should consider couples counseling, while friends should be patient with canceled plans and emotional ups and downs that come with treatment cycles.

Avoiding blame. Don't let anyone carry guilt about infertility. This isn't anyone's fault, and if you're the partner, treatment decisions should be made together rather than placing the burden solely on them.

If you're joining for the visit. If you're the partner, ensure both of you are included in discussions and that testing and treatment burdens are shared fairly. If you're a friend providing support, help them advocate for comprehensive evaluation rather than accepting dismissive responses.

Scenario 20

Same-Sex Family Planning and Single Mother by Choice (SMBC)

Questions to ask, paths to explore, and how to protect your parenthood

You Get to Build This on Purpose

If you're dreaming about building a family, with a partner or on your own, you've probably had to piece it all together from scratch. There's no standard road map for queer parenthood or for becoming a single mother by choice (SMBC). But that's part of what makes this powerful.

You get to do this with intention. You get to ask questions. You get to define your path and protect it.

This guide won't tell you what's right. It will help you prepare for what's next.

What to Expect

Sex ed didn't teach this. There were no whiteboards explaining how two people with uteruses or a single woman could grow a family. No one passed out handouts about donor sperm, reciprocal in vitro fertilization (IVF), or how to pick a clinic that understands your life. If you're here, dreaming about becoming a parent, you probably had to start from scratch with a ton of internet searches. You're not alone.

The good news? While there's more to figure out, there's also opportunity for more intention. You get to build your family on purpose. You get to ask the questions, weigh the options, and design a path that's fully your own.

For many queer couples, the first question is who will carry. Sometimes one person knows they want to be pregnant. Sometimes neither does. Sometimes both do, eventually.

For single parents by choice, the questions can be the same yet different: *Do you want to carry?* What does your body need? How does timing fit into your life? What feels right?

The answers don't have to be immediate or final. They might depend on age, medical history, finances, or just plain desire. That's all okay. There's no quiz. Just a conversation—with yourself or with your partner.

Choosing Your Donor

Most people are surprised by how emotional and logistical this step can be. You can choose a known donor, someone already in your life, or a donor through a sperm bank. Known donors can offer a sense of personal connection, but they require careful planning, clear boundaries, and formal legal agreements before anything moves forward. Medical screening, current sexually transmitted infection testing, and legal protections are essential in these situations and should never be skipped.

Sperm bank donors are medically screened, genetically tested, and legally defined as nonparents, which can offer clarity and peace of mind.

When choosing a donor through a bank, the most important factor is genetic compatibility. You'll undergo expanded carrier screening first, and you'll want a donor who does not carry the same recessive conditions you do. Banks list donors' carrier screening results, medical histories, and often provide audio interviews, photos, essays, or personal details. People often begin with eye color or height but ultimately choose based on a feeling, something about the donor that resonates or feels like a fit for their future family.

Practical considerations matter, too, like whether the donor is identity-release (available to be contacted by the child at age 18), whether there are enough vials available if you want multiple children, and whether the donor's family history aligns with what you feel comfortable with. There's no perfect donor, only the donor that feels right for you.

Understanding Banked Sperm

If you use a sperm bank, the sperm arrives frozen in small vials. What matters most is whether the vial is prepared for use in a clinic or for insemination at home.

Some vials are **washed**, which means the seminal fluid has already been removed. These are used for intrauterine insemination (IUI) in a clinic and are ready to go once thawed.

Other vials are **unwashed** and are typically used for intravaginal or intracervical insemination. Some sperm banks allow these to be used at home if that feels important to you and your partner. Home insemination is usually less effective than IUI, but it can offer privacy, comfort, and the ability to try in your own space without medical intervention.

Both types of vials can also be used for IVF if that becomes part of your plan, though clinics handle any extra preparation.

Considering Clinical Options: Intrauterine Insemination (IUI)

If you're considering clinical options, IUI is often the first stop. It's relatively straightforward: sperm is placed directly into the uterus around ovulation, sometimes with the help of medications like Clomid or Letrozole. You can use a known donor or go through a sperm bank.

This applies equally to couples and single parents building families.

Many clinics have monitoring protocols to help with timing, but not all are set up to support patients who ovulate over the weekend, so that is worth asking in advance. "What do you do if insemination falls on a weekend?" is a fair and telling question.

So is "What's your experience supporting queer couples through this process?" or "What's your experience supporting single parents by choice?"

You'll learn a lot by how they answer. If they hesitate or fumble, if they default to heteronormative language, if they treat your questions like complications—you have every right to look elsewhere. You're not asking for special treatment. You're asking for competent, affirming care.

Home Insemination: Intravaginal Insemination (IVI)

Many queer couples opt for home insemination instead, known as IVI (intravaginal insemination). Many single parents by choice choose this route as well. This can be more intimate and less medicalized.

It's often done with fresh sperm from a known donor, though some banks will ship frozen samples for home use. Timing is everything here, so cycle tracking becomes your best friend.

And while the success rates may be lower than IUI, the emotional experience can be profoundly grounding. It's just you, your partner, your body, your space.

Think Netflix and chill, but with a turkey baster.

And Then There's IVF

IVF is a more intensive path. It involves hormone injections, 8–12 days of monitoring, an egg retrieval under sedation, fertilizing the eggs in the lab, optional genetic testing of embryos, freezing, and ultimately transferring an embryo back into the uterus. IVF can be a first-line choice or a step after other methods haven't worked. It offers higher success rates and more control over timing and embryo quality.

IVF also opens the possibility of reciprocal IVF for couples, where one partner provides the eggs and the other carries the pregnancy, a way for both people to play a role. In addition to fertility reasons, single parents may pursue IVF for reasons like timing, medical factors, or the desire to genetically test embryos. The process can be physically and emotionally demanding, and not all clinics are fully affirming or equipped to support queer families or SMBC, so choosing the right team matters.

Legal Prep for Known Donors

If you're using a known donor, get a written agreement before you begin. It doesn't matter how close you are or how simple everyone thinks the process will be, written terms protect everyone's expectations and ensure that you, not the donor, are the legal parent(s). This step matters for all families and is especially important when you're building a family on your own.

If Pregnancy Isn't Your Path

Some people choose not to pursue pregnancy at all because of health, finances, trauma, timing, or personal preference. Adoption, foster care, and surrogacy are meaningful, valid ways to become a parent. What matters most is working with professionals who immediately recognize your family structure and don't make you justify it on every form or in every conversation.

Why Legal Protection Still Matters

Being listed on a birth certificate is not the same thing as having a court order of parentage. In some states, a birth certificate creates a presumption of parentage, but that presumption can still be challenged, and it is not guaranteed to be recognized if you move, travel, or face a custody dispute. The only fully secure and universally recognized protection is a court order, such as a second-parent adoption or confirmatory parentage order. These orders provide durable legal protection in emergencies, schools, hospitals, and any situation in which your parental relationship may be questioned. It's extra paperwork, but it legally safeguards your family everywhere.

You Don't Need Every Answer Today

If you're thinking about these questions, imagining possibilities, or even just letting yourself want this, you're already moving. You don't have to have the full plan, the perfect timeline, or every decision made. Start with what feels doable: track your cycle, book a consult, read through donor bank FAQs, or look for clinics, agencies, or attorneys who understand the kind of family you're building.

Your path doesn't have to look like anyone else's.

It just has to feel right to you.

Workbook: Thinking Through It

What are you exploring right now?

Check all that apply:

☐ IUI (intrauterine insemination)
☐ Home insemination (IVI)
☐ IVF or reciprocal IVF
☐ Adoption or foster care
☐ Surrogacy
☐ Other: _____

What questions do you want answered?
Use this space to name the information you're still looking for—medical, emotional, logistical, or legal.

_____

_____

_____

What concerns or barriers are showing up?
This could be about your body, your provider, your budget, your timing, or your readiness—whatever feels real.

_____

_____

_____

What would make this feel safe or supportive?
Think about the emotional, medical, financial, or community support you want in place before moving forward.

_____

_____

_____

Planning with a Partner—Whether you're carrying, supporting, or still deciding, use this space to reflect as a team.

Who is exploring carrying (if anyone)?

_____

_____

Are there any medical factors to consider (e.g., endometriosis, fibroids, trauma history)?

_____

_____

What does each person want their role to be in this process—emotionally, physically, or legally?

What path feels most aligned with your goals right now (even if it's just a maybe)?

What is your biggest hope for this process?

What is your biggest fear or hesitation?

What would help you both feel more supported?

SMBC

Why this path? What's drawing you toward single parenthood right now—timing, desire, stability, independence, readiness?

What does support look like for you? Who do you imagine leaning on? Friends, family, community, a doula, a sibling, a therapist? How do you want support to show up?

What feels exciting? What feels overwhelming? Name the parts that feel aligned and the parts that feel heavy or unclear.

_____

_____

What do you need to feel safe? Think about medical care, emotional support, financial planning, legal clarity, or practical help during pregnancy and postpartum.

_____

_____

What's your next step? Track your cycle, schedule a consult, explore donor options, or simply give yourself more space to reflect.

_____

_____

For Support People/Partners

You're building a family while navigating a system that wasn't built for you. The process is emotional, expensive, and often filled with heteronormative assumptions. You both deserve to be seen, supported, and included every step of the way.

Equal involvement. Whether or not you're the one carrying, you're still equal partners. Talk openly about roles, responsibilities, and how to make decisions together. Medically, emotionally, and legally.

Legal protection. Love matters, but paperwork protects. Co-parent adoptions, donor agreements, and legal parentage steps are critical. Don't leave them for later.

Financial planning. This process is often costly. Share the financial load and talk early about expectations, stress points, and limits. Money tensions are real, and naming them helps.

If you're joining for the visit. Watch how you're both treated. Speak up if one of you is sidelined, misgendered, or ignored. You both belong in the room and in this process.

PREGNANCY LOSS AND ABORTION CARE

Scenario 21

Navigating Abortion by Choice

What to ask, how to prepare, and getting the support you need

This section is about ending a pregnancy by choice. Perhaps it's not the right time, not the right circumstance, or not the right path for you. It includes medication abortion (mifepristone and misoprostol, or misoprostol alone), in-clinic procedural abortion, and, in later pregnancies, induction abortion. These are all safe, evidence-based medical options, and millions of people in the United States choose them every year.

But even though abortion is healthcare, it is one of the most contested issues in America. Not because of medicine, but because of politics. The current legal landscape is fragmented and confusing by design. After *Roe v. Wade* fell, every state was left to decide what abortion access looks like within its borders: some states protect it, some restrict it, and others ban it entirely. Court challenges, ballot initiatives, "shield laws," telehealth rules, Federal Drug Administration (FDA) battles over mifepristone, and even digital surveillance concerns shape what care looks like today. And with the possibility of a national ban or federal minimum standard on the horizon, access continues to change, regardless of where you live.

This means your options vary dramatically based on your state, your gestational age, your insurance, and even your ability to travel. At the time of writing, medication abortion can be prescribed via telehealth by providers operating under shield laws and mailed across state lines. However, people living in states hostile to abortion may still face legal risk, and access varies based on location and individual circumstances.

Procedural abortion may be straightforward and quick in one state and nearly impossible to reach in another. Abortion is safe and effective, but the legal landscape is wildly uneven.

You shouldn't have to navigate any of this alone.

Whether you're certain, still deciding, or supporting someone else, you deserve care that is safe, private, and judgment-free. This scenario won't tell you what to choose, that decision belongs to you. What it *will* do is guide you through the practical realities: how medication abortion works, what procedural options look like, what to expect with self-managed care, how to plan for digital privacy, what questions to ask a clinic, and where to turn for legal, financial, and emotional support.

You have options. You have rights. And you deserve care that centers your safety, dignity, and autonomy, no matter where you live.

Medication Abortion versus Procedural Abortion

A clear comparison to help you understand your options. There are two main categories of abortion care in the United States: *medication abortion* and *procedural abortion*. Both are safe, effective, and used every day in clinics across the country. Which one is right for you can depend on how far along the pregnancy is, your health, your preferences, your access to care, and the laws in your state.

Medication Abortion (Including Self-Managed Abortion)

Medication abortion uses FDA-approved pills, mifepristone and misoprostol, to end a pregnancy. It works best in the first trimester and is most commonly used up to 10–12 weeks. Some clinical protocols go up to 12–13 weeks.

How it works:
Medication abortion involves one of two regimens:

1. Mifepristone + misoprostol
Mifepristone blocks progesterone, ending the pregnancy.
Misoprostol, taken 24–48 hours later, causes the uterus to contract and empty.
This method is over 95% effective and is considered the gold standard.

> *Mifepristone has been repeatedly targeted by political attacks. At the time this workbook was written, it is still legal and available, including through mail delivery. Because access can shift, we encourage readers to check the most current information as they move through this workbook.*

2. Misoprostol-only regimen

Misoprostol alone can safely and effectively end a pregnancy (about 85–95% effective).

It requires multiple doses and may take longer, with more cramping and bleeding.

What it feels like:

Most people have strong cramps and heavy bleeding for several hours. Nausea, diarrhea, or chills can happen but usually pass quickly. Bleeding may continue lightly for one to two weeks.

How do I know if it worked:

Most people confirm completion using a high-sensitivity home pregnancy test three to four weeks later. Your clinic may offer a phone follow-up, ultrasound, or blood test if needed. Persistent symptoms, very light bleeding that continues for weeks, or still-positive tests after four weeks may need evaluation.

A small number of people may need an aspiration procedure afterward to complete the abortion or stop heavy bleeding.

Where it can be done:

There are many laws regulating abortion care. Abortion care can happen in several settings depending on the method, your state's laws, and your personal preferences. Some people receive care in a clinic, where providers can offer in-person evaluation, medication, or procedural options. Others use telehealth, which enables you to meet with a clinician virtually and have medication mailed discreetly to your home.

Important. In the United States, *no one should be criminalized for their own abortion*. But people have been investigated for miscarriages and pregnancy outcomes, this is especially concerning when digital trails were misinterpreted or weaponized. This is why digital privacy, secure communication, and knowing your rights matter, especially in states hostile to abortion.

A key fact. If you seek medical care afterward, you do not need to disclose that you are having an abortion or that you have used abortion pills. There is no routine test that can distinguish a medication abortion from a miscarriage. However, vaginal misoprostol may leave visible residue for up to four days, which is why some people choose oral routes if they are concerned about this risk.

When to Seek Emergency Care

Call a clinician, urgent care, or go to the emergency room if you have any of the following:

- Soaking more than *two pads an hour for two hours*
- Fever over 100.4 °F (38 °C) lasting more than 24 hours
- Severe abdominal pain that doesn't improve with pain meds
- Dizziness or fainting
- Foul-smelling discharge

Procedural Abortion

Procedural abortion is a quick, safe in-clinic method performed by trained healthcare professionals. It can be used throughout the first and second trimester, depending on the procedure.

Aspiration abortion (often called D&C in casual language):

- This is used up to about 13–14 weeks.
- The provider gently dilates the cervix and removes the pregnancy with suction.
- It takes about 5–10 minutes, and most people recover within a day or two.

Why people choose this:

- It's fast.
- Bleeding is often lighter afterward.
- You leave the clinic knowing it's complete.
- It can be done later in pregnancy than medication abortion.

Dilation and evacuation (D&E)

- D&Es are used after about 13–14 weeks.
- It involves suction plus instruments to safely empty the uterus.
- Some clinics do it in one day; others over two days.
- Pain control options range from local anesthesia to sedation or general anesthesia.

Induction Abortion

Induction abortion is used later in pregnancy, usually after 14–16 weeks. It uses medications to bring on labor so the pregnancy is delivered, similar to the process of childbirth. It typically occurs in a hospital or specialized facility and can take up to one or two days depending on how a person's body responds.

In some cases, especially in later gestations or depending on state laws and hospital protocols, the care team may recommend an injection (typically digoxin or potassium chloride) to end the pregnancy before labor begins. This step is not always required, varies by setting, and should be explained clearly by your provider so you understand the medical or legal reasons behind it.

Why people choose induction abortion:

- It may be the safest option depending on medical history, fetal diagnosis, or gestational age.
- Some people prefer the option to hold or see the fetus afterward.
- It may be recommended if D&E is unavailable locally.
- It offers a more "labor-like" experience for people who want or need that process.

Comparing the Options in Plain Language

Medication abortion may be right for you if you want privacy, prefer being at home, want to avoid a procedure, or are early in pregnancy. It offers more control and often feels "natural," though cramping and bleeding can be intense and the process takes several hours.

Procedural abortion (D&C or D&E) may be right for you if you want something definitive, want to leave the clinic knowing it's complete, want lighter bleeding at home, or are further along in pregnancy. It's fast, highly effective, and has a short recovery.

Induction abortion may be right for you if you are later in pregnancy, have a medical or fetal indication, or prefer a labor-like process. It usually happens in a hospital, takes many hours to a couple of days, and may include an injection depending on gestational age and local protocols.

Across all three options, abortion remains extremely safe. None affect your future fertility. Each is recognized, evidence-based medical care. You deserve access to the option that fits your needs.

What Is a Crisis Pregnancy Center and How Do I Avoid One?

A crisis pregnancy center, often called a CPC, is a facility that presents itself as a medical clinic or pregnancy resource center but does not provide comprehensive, unbiased reproductive healthcare. These centers are usually anti-abortion and often anti-contraception, and their goal is to discourage people from choosing abortion, sometimes by providing misleading information about pregnancy, abortion, or fertility timelines. They may offer free pregnancy tests or ultrasounds but typically do not provide prenatal care, abortion care, or referrals to licensed providers. To avoid a CPC, look for clinics that clearly list the medical services they provide, including abortion or contraception, confirm that providers are licensed clinicians, and are upfront about costs and options. Tools like ineedana.com, abortionfinder.org, and state abortion funds can help you locate legitimate, evidence-based reproductive healthcare providers.

How to Choose Which Method Is Right for You

Your best option depends on the following considerations:

- How far along the pregnancy is
- What's available in your state and accessible to you
- Your health history
- Whether you can travel or use telehealth
- Your preference for home versus clinic
- Your comfort with pain, privacy, timing, and follow-up
- The legal considerations in your state about medication or self-managed care

Pre-Visit Planning: What to Look For

When calling clinics, ask these questions:

- "What abortion methods do you offer, and up to what gestational age?"
- "What's required before the procedure—waiting periods, multiple visits, and so on?"
- "What are the total costs, and what payment options are available?"
- "Do you provide counseling or support services?"
- "What should I expect on the day of the appointment?"

Red flags to avoid:

- Facilities that won't give clear pricing up front
- Places that seem evasive about their services
- Centers that advertise free services but don't provide medical care
- Any provider that makes you feel judged or pressured

Questions to Ask During Your Visit

Understanding the procedure:

- "Can you walk me through exactly what will happen?"
- "How long will I need to stay here, do I need a driver?"
- "What pain management is available?"

Aftercare and recovery:

- "What should I expect for recovery?"
- "When can I return to normal activities?"
- "When should I call if I have concerns?"
- "How will I know if something's wrong afterward?"
- "What follow-up care is needed?"

Risks and prevention:

- "What are the side effects and risks?"
- "Do you provide birth control, and can I start it today?"

Managing Costs and Access

If cost is a barrier:

- Ask about sliding scale fees or payment plans.
- Look into abortion funds (local and national organizations that help with costs).
- Ask if they accept insurance or Medicaid (where applicable).
- Inquire about reduced-cost days or financial assistance programs.

If you need to travel:

- Factor in transportation, lodging, and time off work.
- Ask if the clinic can coordinate with local support organizations.
- Find out if you'll need multiple visits or if everything can be done in one trip.
- Consider practical support organizations that help with logistics.

Why We Care About Digital Privacy

The laws about abortion access are shifting fast, and in some places digital information—search history, location data, texts—has been used to investigate or question people seeking care. Protecting your digital footprint isn't about paranoia; it's about taking simple steps to keep your health decisions private and under your control.

Digital privacy tips:

- Use a private browser.
- Turn off location services.
- Don't use employer or school devices.
- Delete apps you don't need and clear search history.
- Avoid SMS texting when possible; use Signal if you need to message someone.
- Use period-tracking apps carefully; consider manual tracking.

Workbook: Pre-Decision Reflection

My last known period was: _____

My pregnancy test was positive on: _____

My best guess at how far along I am: _____

Decision-Making Factors

For some, making the decision to have an abortion is simple. For others it's more complex. Use this space to clarify your own thoughts and your plan before seeking care.

This isn't about finding the "right" answer, it's about getting clear on what matters most *to you* in *your* situation. Different factors will carry different weight for different people, and that's completely normal.

For each factor below, ask yourself, *How much does this influence my thinking about this pregnancy?* Then rate it on a scale of 1–5:

- 1 = Not important—This doesn't factor into my decision at all.
- 2 = Slightly important—I've thought about it, but it's not a major consideration.

- 3 = Moderately important—This matters to me and influences my thinking.
- 4 = Very important—This is a significant factor in my decision-making.
- 5 = Extremely important—This is one of the most crucial factors for me.

There are no wrong answers. What matters deeply to one person might be irrelevant to another, and that's okay. The goal is to understand your own priorities so you can make a decision that aligns with what's most important in your life right now.

Factor	Rating (1–5)	Examples	My Thoughts About This?
My physical health		*Am I healthy enough for pregnancy? Do I have conditions that make pregnancy risky?*	
My mental health		*How would pregnancy/parenting affect my depression, anxiety, or other mental health needs?*	
Financial readiness		*Can I afford pregnancy care, birth, and raising a child? How would this affect my financial stability?*	
Relationship status		*Am I in a supportive relationship? How does my partner feel? What if I'm single?*	
Current life goals		*How would this change my plans for the next 5–10 years?*	
Existing children/ family		*How would another child affect the kids I already have? My capacity as a parent?*	
Educational plans		*Am I in school? Would I be able to continue my education?*	
Career considerations		*How would this affect my job, career trajectory, or professional goals?*	
Personal values/ beliefs		*What do my core beliefs tell me? How do my values guide this decision?*	

(continued)

(continued)

Factor	Rating (1–5)	Examples	My Thoughts About This?
Partner's feelings		*What does my partner want? How much should their opinion influence my choice?*	
Family expectations		*What would my family think? How much do their opinions matter to me?*	
Religious considerations		*What does my faith tradition say? How do I balance religious teachings with my personal situation?*	
Timing in my life		*Is this the right time? Would waiting be better? Am I ready now?*	
Age considerations		*Am I too young? Too old? How does my age factor in?*	
Housing stability		*Do I have a stable place to live? Safe housing for a child?*	
Support system		*Who would help me? Do I have people I can rely on?*	
Health insurance		*Can I afford prenatal care and birth? What would healthcare cost?*	
Past pregnancy experiences		*How do previous pregnancies, births, or losses influence this decision?*	
Impact on my body		*How do I feel about the physical changes of pregnancy and birth?*	
Parenting readiness		*Do I want to be a parent? Am I ready for that responsibility?*	
Fear of judgment		*Am I worried about what others will think of my choice?*	
Practical logistics		*Can I get time off work? Transportation to appointments? Childcare for existing kids?*	

After you've gone through this table you might find the following:

- Some factors you thought would matter don't actually influence you much.
- Other considerations feel more important than you expected.
- Your ratings help clarify what's really driving your feelings about this decision.
- It's easier to see which factors are emotional versus practical versus value-based.

After you rate everything, look for patterns:

- Which factors got 4s and 5s? These are your key considerations to help you right now.
- Are your highest-rated factors mostly practical, emotional, or value-based?
- Do your ratings point toward a particular decision, or do they feel conflicted?
- What would happen if you only considered your top three factors?

This exercise isn't meant to make the decision for you. It's meant to help you find clarity and understand what's important to you so that whatever you decide feels truly aligned with your values and circumstances.

For Support People

They're making a personal decision about pregnancy while potentially facing judgment, legal barriers, and logistical challenges. They need unconditional support for their choice, not your opinions about what they "should" do.

Supporting their autonomy. This is their decision to make. Your job is to support them, not influence their choice in either direction.

Practical assistance. Help with transportation, childcare, time off work, and recovery logistics without making them feel like a burden.

Emotional presence. Follow their lead on how much they want to talk about the experience. Some people process by talking, others need space.

Different support roles. If you're their partner, you may have complex feelings about the pregnancy and other decisions that need processing—but not with them right now. Find your own support system to work through your emotions so you can show up fully for theirs. If you're a friend, your role is clearer: provide practical and emotional support without judgment. Both roles require putting their needs first during this vulnerable time.

Managing your own feelings. Whether you're partner or friend, you might feel sadness, relief, anxiety, or confusion about their choice. These feelings are valid but shouldn't become their burden to manage. Process your emotions separately so you can offer genuine, unconditional support.

If you're joining for the visit. Support their decision and help ensure they receive respectful, nonjudgmental care. If you're the partner, don't use the appointment to express your own feelings about the pregnancy or decision.

Scenario 22

Termination for Medical Reasons (TFMR)

When a wanted pregnancy faces serious medical complications—
navigating an impossible decision with compassion and support

Before You Begin

Termination for medical reasons (TFMR) refers to ending a pregnancy because of a medical diagnosis affecting the fetus, the pregnant person, or both. It is not a decision anyone expects to face. TFMR most often occurs in deeply wanted pregnancies, when parents are preparing for a baby and instead are confronted with devastating medical news.

Often, TFMR comes after an abnormal ultrasound, a genetic finding, or a sudden medical complication. One day all seems well with the pregnancy, and the next you're being asked to learn complex medical terminology, meet with specialists, and make quick decisions under emotional shock.

TFMR carries a unique kind of grief. You are not simply making a medical choice; you are mourning the loss of a future you thought you were building. And because the US healthcare system is fragmented, TFMR care can feel even harder, especially in states where abortion restrictions delay or deny needed care.

You deserve a team that honors your grief, respects this pregnancy, and supports you with clarity and compassion.

Understanding What Happened: Diagnosis Pathways

When facing TFMR, one of the hardest parts is understanding *where* the information came from and *how certain* it is. Most people learn about these tests for the first time in crisis, and the language, *"abnormal." "high risk," "incompatible with life,"* cans sound definitive while actually meaning very different things medically.

Many TFMR decisions are made only after diagnostic testing confirms what screening tests first suggested. Here's what each test actually provides:

Ultrasound findings:
- Ultrasound may show structural differences (brain, heart, kidneys, spine), growth concerns, or abnormal fluid patterns.
- It can strongly *suggest* a problem, but doesn't always tell you how severe it is or why it happened.

Noninvasive prenatal testing (NIPT)—screening, not diagnosis:
- NIPT looks at placental DNA in your bloodstream. A positive result means *increased risk*, not certainty.
- It can have false positives and false negatives, especially for rare conditions.
- Screening = "This *might* be a problem."

Chorionic villus sampling (CVS)—diagnostic:
- This test is done about 10–13 weeks.
- CVS analyzes placental cells and can confirm many chromosomal conditions, though results can occasionally be complicated by placental differences.

Amniocentesis—diagnostic:
- This test is typically done after 15 weeks.
- Amnio tests fetal cells directly from the amniotic fluid and is the gold standard for genetic diagnosis.

Maternal health complications:
- Sometimes the medical indication is about the pregnant person's health, not the fetus.

Screening Versus Diagnosis: Why It Matters

In these moments, you need clarity, not vague language like *abnormal* or *concerning*.

Screening tests (like NIPT and some ultrasounds) can do the following:
- Estimate risk
- Cannot confirm anything
- Should be followed by diagnostic testing whenever possible

Diagnostic tests (CVS and amnio):
- Confirm or rule out conditions
- Provide the most accurate information for decision-making

The one question that cuts through everything: "Is this a screening or diagnosis? How certain are we?" You deserve clear answers, real numbers, and explanations you can understand.

Seeking Specialized Care—Finding Providers for TFMR

Because abortion care is restricted in many states, accessing care for TFMR often requires referral to a maternal fetal medicine (MFM) specialist, an abortion clinic that provides care at later gestational ages, or a hospital willing and able to perform induction termination. Not all general OB-GYNs provide abortion care, and many are legally or institutionally restricted from doing so, which means referrals can be delayed or incomplete. Knowing that specialized care is often required can help you advocate for timely referrals and avoid unnecessary roadblocks during an already stressful time.

Questions to ask when calling clinics or MFMs:
- "Do you provide TFMR at ___ weeks gestation?"
- "What's your experience with this specific diagnosis?"
- "Do you offer genetic counseling as part of care?"
- "What are the options at this gestational age: D&E, induction, or both?"
- "If we choose induction, can we see or hold the baby?"
- "Do you provide footprints, photos, or memory items?"
- "Is pastoral care or bereavement support available if I desire that?"

Red flags:

- Evasive answers about gestational age
- Language that minimizes your grief
- Providers who seem rushed or judgmental
- Any clinic unable to clearly articulate what they offer

Processing the News: Decision-Making in Crisis

When you receive a life-altering diagnosis in pregnancy, sometimes your brain goes into survival mode. Shock, fear, grief, and information overload can make it nearly impossible to think clearly, let alone make a medical decision. This chart is here to help you slow things down and separate the emotions, the facts, and the practical realities so you can understand what's influencing you most.

This is *not* a quiz and it's not meant to point you toward a "right" answer. It's simply a tool to help you organize your thoughts during a moment when everything feels chaotic. By rating each factor, you're able to see what's weighing heaviest on your heart and what concerns may be less central than you expected. Many parents find that putting numbers to these questions brings clarity, reveals patterns, or makes it easier to talk through the decision with a partner or provider.

Use the following table in whatever way feels most supportive: alone, with a partner, or during a counseling session. The goal is not to justify your decision to anyone else. The goal is to understand *your own priorities*, so that whatever choice you make is grounded in your values, your reality, and your love for this pregnancy.

Rate how important each factor is in your decision-making: (1 = not important, 5 = extremely important) and add your thoughts in the table.

Factor	Rating (1–5)	Examples	My Thoughts About This
Severity of diagnosis		*How serious is the condition? Is it incompatible with life?*	
Quality-of-life concerns		*What would life look like for this child? Pain, suffering, medical interventions?*	
Medical risks to me		*Does continuing pregnancy threaten my health or life?*	

Factor	Rating (1–5)	Examples	My Thoughts About This
Impact on existing children		*How would intensive caregiving affect my other kids?*	
Long-term caregiving capacity		*Am I emotionally, physically, financially prepared for complex medical needs?*	
Partner's feelings/ alignment		*Are we united in this decision?*	
Certainty of diagnosis		*How confident are the doctors? Is there room for error?*	
Timing/gestational age		*How does being further along affect my options and feelings?*	
Family support system		*Who would help with intensive care needs long-term?*	
Religious/spiritual beliefs		*How do my beliefs guide me through this decision?*	
Previous loss experience		*How do past pregnancy losses influence my thinking?*	
Financial considerations		*Can we afford lifetime medical care, therapies, equipment?*	
My mental health		*How am I coping with this? What do I need?*	
Hope for treatment/ cure		*Is research advancing? Could future treatments help?*	

The three most important factors for me are the following:

1. _____

2. _____

3. _____

Understanding Your Medical Options

Your options for TFMR depend on gestational age, the diagnosis, your medical history, and the laws in your state. In early pregnancy, medication abortion may be an option, though it is less commonly used in TFMR because many diagnoses occur later. In the second trimester and beyond, dilation and evacuation (D&E) or induction abortion become the primary forms of care. Each option carries different medical, emotional, and logistical considerations. There is no "easy" choice, only the one that best fits your needs, your values, and your circumstances.

Dilation and evacuation (D&E) is typically offered starting about 13–14 weeks. It is a brief procedure with a shorter physical recovery and is often the safest option when the pregnant person's health is at risk. However, access varies widely, as some hospitals, health systems, and states do not offer D&E.

Induction abortion is more commonly used later in pregnancy, often after 16 weeks, or when families prefer a labor-like experience. This option keeps the fetus intact, which may allow families to see, hold, photograph, or create memory items if they choose.

In some cases, particularly with later induction abortions, families may elect to have a feticidal injection beforehand. This option is not always easily available and may require referral to a specialized provider, additional appointments, travel, and significant out-of-pocket cost. For some families, these logistical and financial barriers can make this option inaccessible or prohibitive. When this is part of the conversation, providers should clearly explain why it is being offered or required, what it involves, and what alternatives exist within the constraints of local law and hospital policy.

In rare, emergent situations, such as severe infection, organ failure, or other life-threatening complications, additional interventions may be recommended. Your medical team should explain why these options are necessary and what they mean for your safety, care, and recovery.

Questions to ask about the procedure. When you're trying to understand what each option would actually look and feel like, ask these questions:

- "Can you explain exactly what this procedure involves?"
- "How long will the process take from start to finish?"
- "What kind of anesthesia or pain management is available?"
- "If I want to, will I be able to see or hold the baby afterward?"
- "What are the risks, and what should I expect physically afterward?"
- "How many days will I likely need off work to recover?"

Questions to ask about aftercare. After the procedure, you deserve clear guidance on what comes next. Ask these questions:

- "Will my milk come in, and how will we manage lactation suppression?"
- "What follow-up care do you recommend? Medical, mental health, or both?"
- "If we want to get pregnant again, when is it safe to try?"
- "Can you provide documentation for work or family leave?"

Pre-Visit Planning

When you're facing TFMR, the emotional weight often overshadows the practical details, but these logistics matter and this workbook exists to support you. Planning ahead can create a small sense of stability during a time that feels anything but stable. Use this section to map out what you'll need financially, logistically, and emotionally so that the day of the procedure feels as supported as possible.

Financial and logistical considerations. Even with insurance, TFMR can come with unexpected expenses: travel, missed work, hotel stays, childcare, or out-of-pocket charges. Outline what you know now, and fill in the rest as you get more information.

Support I want to have the day of the procedure and the days that follow:

_____

What I want to bring for comfort (clothes, blanket, music, snacks, etc.):

_____

Memorial or remembrance. Not everyone wants to think about memory-making right now—and that's okay. But for many families, having the option matters later, even if they don't choose it in the moment. This space helps you note what feels right for you today, knowing it may change.

Memorial or remembrance plans I'm considering:

- ☐ Footprints or handprints   ☐ Photos   ☐ Naming the baby
- ☐ Small memorial or ceremony   ☐ Burial and tombstone
- ☐ Keepsake jewelry   ☐ Planting something in memory
- ☐ Donation to a relevant charity   ☐ I'm not ready to think about this yet
- ☐ Other: _____

What's Often Missing from TFMR Counseling

TFMR care is often medically thorough but emotionally incomplete. Many parents leave the hospital or clinic with more questions than answers because the system focuses heavily on the procedure and far less on the physical and emotional realities that come afterward. These are the pieces that should be standard in TFMR counseling, but too often are not.

Lactation Suppression

If your TFMR occurs in the second or third trimester, your milk may come in afterward. This can be a deeply painful experience for many parents, especially if unexpected. This is a normal physiologic response to pregnancy hormones and has nothing to do with your choices or the circumstances of your loss. Providers don't always prepare families for this, leaving people blindsided. You deserve clear guidance before it happens, including whether your care team can prescribe medication like cabergoline (if medically appropriate), or provide instructions for non-medication approaches such as compression, ice, nonsteroidal anti-inflammatory drugs, and avoiding stimulation. A simple question "Will you help me prevent lactation and explain what to expect?" can save you days of physical and emotional distress.

Chromosomal and Genetic Testing Options

Families facing TFMR often want answers, about what happened and what it means for future pregnancies, but these options are not always explained. Depending on your gestational age and the procedure you choose, fetal or placental testing may still be possible. This can include karyotype, microarray, pathology, or other specialized studies that help clarify whether a condition was random, inherited, or likely to recur. Ask your care team, "Can testing be done after delivery or D&E, what type do you recommend, and how will the results guide our future pregnancies?" Even when results don't change the outcome, they can provide a sense of understanding, closure, or direction for the future.

Follow-Up Mental Health Support

TFMR grief is different from miscarriage grief, different from stillbirth grief, and different from elective abortion grief. It blends trauma, shock, love, guilt, heartbreak, and medical fear in ways that most general pregnancy-loss spaces aren't equipped to hold.

Many parents benefit from trauma-informed therapy, TFMR-specific support groups, and guidance tailored to future pregnancies, which often come with heightened anxiety and complex emotions. This support is not optional, it is part of comprehensive care. If your provider does not bring it up, ask, "Do you have referrals for TFMR-informed therapy or support groups, and what mental health resources are available as we navigate this?" You deserve support that honors both your grief and the love you carried into this pregnancy.

Planning for Future Pregnancies

This is one of the most overlooked parts of TFMR care and one of the most important. Many parents leave the hospital without guidance about what comes next. But follow-up care, recurrence counseling, and future pregnancy planning should be standard. Your care team should walk you through what to expect medically and emotionally as you think ahead. These questions can guide your follow-up visits, especially if you're considering another pregnancy:

- "Do we need genetic counseling before trying again?"
- "What would monitoring look like in a future pregnancy?"
- "How long should we wait before trying to conceive?"
- "What are the chances this could happen again?"
- "What support is available during a subsequent pregnancy?"

As you find your way through this, keep this close:

What you're feeling is real and what you lost is significant. You made a decision rooted in love, responsibility, care, and perhaps foresight. Healing doesn't happen all at once, give yourself permission to move at your own pace. Honor this pregnancy in whatever way feels right, and let yourself grow around the grief rather than through it.

Carry what you need forward. Leave what you can behind.

Though it may feel like it, you are not walking this path alone.

For Support People

They're facing a devastating loss of a wanted pregnancy and making impossible decisions about their baby's suffering and their family's future. They need someone who understands there are many layers and nuances to this decision.

Honoring the loss. This was a wanted baby who was loved. Acknowledge their grief and don't minimize the loss because of the circumstances, but let them set the tone for what they need.

Supporting decisions. Trust that they're making the most loving decision possible in an impossible situation. Don't second-guess their choice.

Long-term grief. This loss may affect them for years. Remember important dates and don't expect them to "move on" according to anyone else's timeline.

Different support roles. If you're their partner, you're grieving the same loss while also supporting them through the medical process. Your grief matters, too, but you may need to process some of it separately so you can also be present for their needs. If you're a friend or family member, understand that this is a profound loss and they may need the compassionate, long-term support.

Managing your own grief. Whether you're a partner or friend, you may feel overwhelming sadness, anger at the unfairness, or helplessness about the situation. These feelings are normal and valid. Find your own grief support so you can show up for their mourning process without adding the burden of managing your emotions to their already overwhelming experience.

If you're going to the visit too. Help them process complex medical information and support their decision-making without adding pressure. Pay attention and take notes, this experience is so overwhelming for them that having someone who remembers the medical details, timing, and next steps is incredibly valuable.

Scenario 23

Selective Reduction in Multifetal Pregnancy

What it means, how it's performed, and how to process both the physical and emotional layers of the decision

Bringing new life into the world doesn't always go as planned. Sometimes, it brings unexpected abundance: two, three, or even more heartbeats flickering on the screen. For some, that moment comes after years of fertility treatment; for others, it happens spontaneously, without any intervention at all. Either way, the emotions can be complicated: excitement, shock, fear, awe, gratitude, and panic often live side by side.

Multifetal pregnancy and reduction is rarely discussed and even more rarely supported, despite being a well-established part of reproductive healthcare. Selective or multifetal reduction is a medical procedure used to reduce the number of fetuses in a multifetal pregnancy in order to protect the pregnant person's health and improve the chances of a safer pregnancy and delivery. It is not about taking away a pregnancy. It is about making a medically complex pregnancy more survivable for both the pregnant person and the remaining fetuses.

When your doctor first mentions reduction, it might feel like the ground drops out from under you. You may find yourself thinking, *How did we get here? Why me? How do I even begin to make this decision?* These are normal questions and there are no easy answers. But you deserve full information, compassionate care, and the space to process every piece of what this means.

Or maybe you thought about reduction yourself before anyone else said it out loud. Maybe you've already played out the scenarios in your head, wondering what kind of parent that makes you. You are *not* a bad parent for thinking about safety, limits, or survival. You are not selfish for wanting to protect your body, your health, your family, or the babies you hope to bring home.

This section exists because there aren't enough spaces that acknowledge what this decision really feels like: the quiet grief, the fear, the logic, the love. It's here to give language, context, and care to something that too many people face in silence. It's here to remind you that you deserve care that meets you where you are, even in the hardest gray areas of medicine.

Why It's Considered

Carrying multiples increases the risks for both the pregnant person and the fetuses. These risks can include the following:

- **Severe preterm birth** (before 32 weeks), leading to neonatal intensive care unit (NICU) stays or long-term complications
- **Maternal health risks** such as preeclampsia, gestational diabetes, hemorrhage, or heart strain
- **Fetal growth restriction** in which one or more babies do not get adequate nutrients or oxygen
- **Loss of the entire pregnancy** due to complications of multiple gestation
- **Structural or genetic abnormalities** in one fetus that endanger the others

Reduction is not a decision taken lightly. It's a medically guided process designed to balance complex risks, protecting your health and improving the chances for the remaining fetuses.

Preparing for the Decision

You don't have to have all the answers right away. Start by getting all the *information*. Ask for a detailed explanation of these facts:

- The medical reasoning behind recommending reduction
- The risks of continuing versus reducing

- The number of fetuses, their positions, and whether they share a placenta or amniotic sac
- What outcomes your doctor expects for you and the remaining fetuses

If possible, *request a separate counseling session*. You're entitled to time, clarity, and emotional support before making this choice.

Questions to Ask

- "Can you explain why you're recommending reduction in my specific case?"
- "What are the potential outcomes if we continue as is?"
- "What are the risks for my health if I carry all fetuses?"
- "How experienced is this facility or team with performing reductions?"
- "What does the procedure entail, step-by-step, in plain language?"
- "What should I expect physically afterward? Bleeding, cramping, activity limits?"
- "What warning signs mean I should call or come in?"
- "What does aftercare look like?"
- "Can I talk with a mental health provider or counselor familiar with selective reduction?"
- "Will future ultrasounds show anything related to the reduction, and how will you talk me through that?"

Scripts for Self-Advocacy

- "I need to understand both the medical and emotional sides of this before deciding."
- "Please walk me through what the procedure will look like and how I'll feel afterward."
- "I'd like to know how you'll support me physically and emotionally after this procedure."
- "I want to make a decision based on facts, not fear. Please be direct with me about risks and options."
- And it's okay to say: "I may need information repeated or slowed down. This is a lot to process."

What the Procedure Involves

Most multifetal reductions are performed between 11 and 14 weeks of pregnancy by a maternal–fetal medicine (MFM) specialist. The procedure is done under continuous ultrasound guidance, using local anesthesia or light sedation. You'll likely arrive early, have bloodwork or a brief ultrasound, and meet with the doctor and counselor beforehand to review the plan and ask any last questions.

During the procedure, the MFM specialist uses a very thin needle, guided by ultrasound, to deliver a medication that safely stops cardiac activity in the selected fetus. This part is precise, deliberate, and often far less climactic than people expect. The reduction itself usually takes 20–60 minutes from start to finish.

Afterward, you'll be monitored for several hours and may go home the same day. Cramping, light bleeding, and fatigue are normal for a few days. A follow-up ultrasound is typically scheduled within the week to ensure the pregnancy remains stable.

Even with medical clarity, the emotional experience can be profound. Many people describe the day as *quiet, surreal,* or *numb.* Others remember flashes of tenderness—partners holding hands, doctors speaking softly, nurses who made eye contact and didn't look away.

What Happens After the Procedure

After the injection, the selected fetus will no longer grow. Over the next several weeks, the tissue gradually becomes smaller and flatter, a natural process called resorption or *fetal papyraceous.* This doesn't cause physical pain or symptoms, and most people won't feel anything different as it happens. On future ultrasounds, you may see a thin, compressed sac, or you may see very little at all; by the third trimester, the tissue is often difficult to distinguish. The reduced fetus is usually delivered along with the placenta at birth, with no additional procedures needed. Meanwhile, the remaining fetus or fetuses continue to grow normally, and your care shifts to close monitoring with your MFM team. Medically, the goal is to protect the ongoing pregnancy. Emotionally, this part of the journey can be just as complex as the decision itself. Carrying both loss and hope in the same body, at the same time. Nothing about that duality means you made the wrong choice. It means you are human, and navigating something profoundly hard with as much love and clarity as you can.

Pros and Cons to Help You Think Through the Decision

This list is not here to tell you what to do or to push you toward any one choice. It exists to help you see your thoughts and feelings reflected on the page. Sometimes naming what you're carrying makes it feel a little less heavy. You may recognize yourself in one line, many lines, or different lines on different days. That's normal. Circle what resonates. Ignore what doesn't. Come back to this as often as you need. This is about feeling seen, understood, and less alone as you move through a decision that is deeply personal and uniquely yours.

Potential Benefits/Pros	Possible Challenges/Cons
Reduces significant health risks to the pregnant person	Emotional complexity—grief, guilt, and relief may coexist
Improves the chances of a healthy, full-term pregnancy	Limited public understanding; may feel stigmatized or isolating
Decreases the risk of NICU stays and complications for surviving babies	Physical reminders (bleeding, ultrasounds) can be emotionally triggering.
Enables more individualized care and monitoring for remaining fetuses	May conflict with cultural, spiritual, or family beliefs
Protects long-term fertility and future pregnancies	Heightened anxiety for the remainder of the pregnancy
Brings the pregnancy into alignment with family planning goals and personal capacity after birth (emotional, physical, financial)	Navigating conversations with others—especially loved ones who may not understand the decision
May allow for more focused bonding and recovery in the postpartum period	Feelings of guilt or what-if thoughts resurfacing later in pregnancy or after delivery

Your reflections: *(Use the space below to write or circle your top priorities.)*

What risks or values feel most important to you right now?

_____

What outcomes matter most—to your body, your health, your family, your heart?

_____

Processing the Emotional Layers

This experience is often described as *lonely*. Few people even know about selective reduction, let alone talk about it. It can be difficult to explain to others, especially in a culture that divides pregnancy into "good" or "bad," "wanted" or "unwanted." Reduction doesn't fit neatly into those boxes.

You may feel deep love for the pregnancy you're continuing and grief for the one you're not. You might feel protective, angry, numb, or grateful—all at once. All of those feelings are valid.

If you conceived after infertility or pregnancy loss, the guilt can cut even deeper: *I fought so hard to get here, how can I end part of it?*

But choosing reduction is not an act of rejection. It's an act of protection. An act of honoring your limits, your health, and the babies who remain.

If it helps, consider creating a private ritual of acknowledgment:

- Write a letter or journal about the decision.
- Light a candle or plant something in memory.
- Name or symbolically honor the fetus(es) you reduced.
- Schedule time with a therapist or support group afterward.

Grief after reduction is real and worthy of care. You don't have to minimize it just because your pregnancy continues.

What This Might Sound Like in Real Life

"I knew what I could handle, but that didn't make it easy. I loved all of them—but I also knew I needed to make a choice that kept me, and the rest of my family, safe."

"Everyone tells you to just be grateful to be pregnant. But no one talks about what happens when gratitude and fear collide. I made the decision with my head, but I still had to grieve with my heart."

"For me, it came down to capacity—what I could manage physically, emotionally, and after birth. It wasn't about giving up; it was about making sure the babies/baby I could carry had the best chance."

These reflections aren't here to convince you of anything. They're here so you don't feel alone in something that's rarely spoken aloud. Real people say these things when they finally feel safe enough to tell the truth about what this decision actually feels like: the mix of love, fear, clarity, and grief that can live in the same breath. Hearing their words can help you recognize yourself in someone else's experience, remind you that your feelings are valid in all their complexity, and show you that making a medically necessary choice doesn't negate love or hope. These voices exist to sit beside you, not guide you. Here to help so you have language and companionship while navigating something no one ever imagines facing.

Reflection and Journaling Prompts

What emotions are most present for you right now?
(List as many as come up: anger, guilt, relief, sadness, gratitude, confusion, peace.)

___

What do you need most from your care team in the next few weeks?
(Support, reassurance, space, information, validation.)

___

How can you honor both the loss and the continuation of this pregnancy?
(Small rituals, shared conversations, or private reflections.)

___

What words or reminders bring you comfort when the guilt or sadness resurfaces?
(Examples: "I made this choice out of love." "I am protecting the life that remains." "Two things can be true.")

___

For Support People

They're facing a profound and complicated crossroads. Carrying love for the family they imagined and making a decision to protect their health, their future, and the baby or babies who remain. This is not a simple loss, and not a simple choice. They need people around them who understand that this decision lives in the gray, where love, fear, grief, and survival all intersect.

Honor the complexity. This was likely a wanted pregnancy, and reduction doesn't erase that. Acknowledge the grief without minimizing it or trying to make it tidy. Let them decide how much they want to share, and follow their lead on language, pacing, and tone.

Support the decision, don't lean into debate. They've made the most informed and loving choice possible in an impossible situation. Don't question whether they "could have managed" or "should have tried." Trust their medical team, trust their capacity, and trust them.

Be steady in the long arc of grief. People often grieve the reduced fetus quietly and privately, sometimes long after the rest of the world has moved on. Remember important dates, check in gently, and understand that the grief can resurface during ultrasounds, delivery, birthdays, or seemingly out of nowhere.

Understand your role. If you're the partner, your grief matters, too, but you may need to process some of it separately so you can be present for the physical and emotional demands they're carrying. If you're a friend or family member, know that your steadiness, presence, and nonjudgment mean more than perfect words.

Manage your own emotions separately. It's normal to feel sad, overwhelmed, or helpless watching someone you love move through this. Get support for your feelings so you're not asking them to take care of your grief on top of their own.

If you're attending appointments. Your job is to be a calm anchor. Take notes, ask clarifying questions if they freeze, and help them remember the medical details. Sit beside them without rushing, without trying to fix it, and without adding pressure. This moment is already heavy. Your presence should feel like a hand steadying their back, not a weight on their shoulders.

Scenario 24

Miscarriage Management

What to say, what to ask for, and how to advocate when care is delayed or denied (includes scripts for when you're told to "just wait it out")

D espite being incredibly common, occurring in roughly one out of every four pregnancies, miscarriage is still surrounded by silence, stigma, and a long history of minimization. For generations, people were expected to endure pregnancy loss privately, returning to daily life without acknowledgment or support. That legacy lingers today. Many hesitate to talk about their loss for fear of being judged, dismissed, or blamed. And woven through our culture is a quiet superstition: don't talk about miscarriage, don't ask about it, don't prepare for it. Almost as if acknowledging the possibility might invite it. Because of that, most people have no idea what to expect until they're in the middle of it. Then comes the scramble: What is normal bleeding? What isn't? How much pain is too much? When do I need help? And will the system take me seriously?

Too often, the medical system makes an already painful situation even harder. Emergency rooms (ERs) aren't designed for reproductive emergencies unless they are imminently life-threatening. People may sit in waiting rooms for hours while bleeding heavily or experiencing severe pain. They may be sent home with vague instructions like "come back if it gets worse," with little explanation of what "worse" actually means—physically or emotionally. Miscarriage can leave people isolated and unsure, trying to navigate medical uncertainty at the same moment they're processing loss.

This section is here to guide you through it. Whether you're still bleeding, waiting for test results, being told to "watch and wait," or simply trying to understand what just happened, this guide is for you. It won't fix the broken system, but it can give you the clarity, language, and support you deserve when care falls short.

How Did We Get Here? Why Miscarriage Management Is Broken

Miscarriage care has been inadequate for decades. Long before *Dobbs v. Jackson Women's Health Organization*, patients were sent home with "rest and fluids," left to bleed through their clothes, told everything was "fine" when it wasn't, or forced to navigate loss with little information and even less support. Culturally, miscarriage has been treated as a private sorrow. Something people were expected to endure quietly, without burdening anyone else. Medically, it was seen as routine, and anything "routine" is rarely treated with the urgency or compassion it deserves.

But abortion bans have made an already broken system dangerous.

The same treatments used for elective abortion and procedures like dilation and curettage (D&C)—are also the safest, most effective treatments for miscarriage. When those tools become legally restricted, politically weaponized, or poorly understood, miscarriage care gets caught in the crossfire. Providers become fearful. Pharmacies hesitate. Hospitals create unnecessary hoops. And patients are left waiting, sometimes for hours, sometimes for days, while their bodies are actively miscarrying.

Add to all of this the long-standing stigma surrounding pregnancy loss and the quiet superstition that talking about miscarriage might somehow "tempt fate," and you get a system where people desperately need information, but rarely receive it ahead of time. Clinicians rarely talk about miscarriage unless it's already happening, which means patients are trying to process complex medical decisions in the middle of fear, pain, and shock. And now, in a post-*Dobbs* landscape, where miscarriage and abortion treatments overlap, many clinicians are unsure, or afraid, to provide timely, appropriate care.

Let's Start with the Language

The language around miscarriage is limited. And that's exactly why it matters. These terms aren't here to confuse you; they reveal a truth most people were never taught: *miscarriage care and abortion care are not separate worlds. They rely on the same physiology, the same medications, the same procedures, and the same clinicians.* We are in this crisis because lawmakers have decided those overlaps are grounds for restriction, fear, and punishment.

Here's what the medical terms actually mean:

- **Spontaneous abortion.** This is the clinical term for a miscarriage that happens naturally. It describes what your body is doing on its own.
- **Missed abortion.** The pregnancy has stopped developing, but your body hasn't passed the tissue yet. Many people have no symptoms; it's often discovered on ultrasound and may require medication or a procedure.
- **Incomplete abortion.** Some, but not all, pregnancy tissue has passed. This can cause prolonged bleeding or infection risk and also may require medication or a procedure.

These terms can feel surprising because our culture treats "abortion" as something radically different from miscarriage. But medically, they are part of the *same continuum of care.*

That's the point: *you cannot separate miscarriage management from abortion care.*

The body doesn't. Medicine doesn't. Only politics does. And that political separation is why miscarriage care is suffering.

The safest, most effective medications for miscarriage—mifepristone and misoprostol—are the same medications used for abortion. But mifepristone is so tightly regulated and so politically targeted that many clinicians won't prescribe it at all, even though it should be standard care. They fear legal consequences, pharmacy refusals, and institutional scrutiny.

So instead of receiving evidence-based care, patients are told to wait. To pass tissue on their own. To come back later. To endure days or weeks of bleeding, uncertainty, and pain. *Not because it's medically necessary, but because abortion has been criminalized.*

This is the connection everyone needs to understand:

- When abortion access is restricted, miscarriage care is restricted.
- When clinicians fear providing abortion care, they fear providing miscarriage care.
- When lawmakers attack abortion medication, they attack miscarriage management.
- When we lose abortion rights, patients losing wanted pregnancies are the first to suffer.

And here's why this matters for you right now: *When you understand that miscarriage care is abortion care, you can recognize when you're being denied appropriate treatment—and you can learn to advocate for what your body needs in the moment.* You don't have to accept delays, dismissals, or "just wait and see" when better, safer options exist.

Miscarriage is not a crime. It is a medical event that deserves timely, compassionate care—and abortion bans have gotten in the way.

Your Management Options—A Quick Overview

Depending on your symptoms, how far along the pregnancy was, and your preferences, miscarriage is usually managed in one of three ways:

- **Expectant management (wait and see).** Letting the miscarriage progress naturally. This can take days or weeks and may involve unpredictable bleeding and cramping. Some people prefer this approach because it avoids medication or surgery. Others find the uncertainty exhausting.
- **Medication management.** Taking misoprostol (sometimes with mifepristone) to help your body pass the pregnancy. Expect bleeding, cramping, and the passage of tissue within hours to days. This option offers more control than waiting, but without the need for surgery.
- **Surgical management.** A brief procedure in a clinic or hospital, such as a D&C, to remove pregnancy tissue. This choice is picked for many reasons: safety, closure, speed, or if other options haven't worked.

All three are valid. And you should have the ability to choose what works for you. You deserve accurate information, enough time to ask questions, and care that treats you like more than a checklist.

Miscarriage Management Options: Side-by-Side Comparison

Category	Expectant Management ("Wait and See")	Medication Management (Misoprostol ± Mifepristone)	Procedural Management (D&C or Manual Vacuum Aspiration)
Why someone might choose it	• Want to avoid meds or procedures • Feels more comfortable letting the body do this naturally • No urgent medical red flags	• Want more control and a clearer timeline • Prefer to avoid surgery • Comfortable managing bleeding/pain at home with support	• Want fastest, most predictable option • Need or want completion in a single visit • Heavy bleeding, anemia, infection concerns, or failure of other methods

Category	Expectant Management ("Wait and See")	Medication Management (Misoprostol ± Mifepristone)	Procedural Management (D&C or Manual Vacuum Aspiration)
What it's like	• Bleeding/cramping that comes and goes over **days to weeks** • Timing is unpredictable • Typically requires follow-up ultrasound	• Pills taken at home or in clinic • Heavy bleeding/cramping within hours • Passing clots/tissue (often intense but short-lived) • May need a second dose	• Brief procedure (minutes) in clinic/operating room • Local anesthesia or sedation • Light bleeding afterward • Most people back to normal activity in one to two days
Main risks/challenges	• Heavy or prolonged bleeding • Incomplete miscarriage (may still need meds/procedure) • Infection if tissue remains • Emotional strain from waiting/not knowing	• Intense cramping + gastrointestinal symptoms (nausea, chills, diarrhea) • Incomplete miscarriage (may still need procedure)	• Low infection risk • Very small risk of uterine perforation or scarring (higher with sharp curettage) • Emotional impact of undergoing a procedure • Cost
What to watch for/when to call	• Soaking a pad in less than one to two hours • Dizziness, faintness, racing heart • Fever or chills • Severe one-sided pain • Foul-smelling discharge	• Soaking pads rapidly for more than a couple hours • Very large clots with dizziness or weakness • Fever lasting > 24 hours after meds • Severe pain not relieved by meds • Anything that makes you feel unsafe	• Bleeding heavier than a period for more than a few hours • Fever/chills • Worsening pain instead of improvement • Foul discharge

Questions to ask when you're miscarrying:

- "What are my options right now: expectant, medication, or surgical?"
- "What risks should I watch for at home?"
- "What pain relief can I have here—and what should I take later?"
- "Was my human chorionic gonadotropin level tested? What was it, and how will we track it?"
- "How will I know when the miscarriage is complete?"
- "Do I need a follow-up visit or more bloodwork?"
- "Do I need to wait before trying to get pregnant again?"
- "Can we talk about what this means for future pregnancies?"

Genetic Testing

Genetic testing of the pregnancy tissue can sometimes help answer the question everyone asks after miscarriage: "Why did this happen?" Testing can identify chromosomal causes of the loss, which is most useful if you've had more than one miscarriage, are over 35, or are planning future fertility treatment like in vitro fertilization. It won't predict whether you can get pregnant again, and it won't prevent another miscarriage, but sometimes it can offer clarity. This option is available with a D&C and, in some cases, with tissue passed at home if you're given a container and instructions in advance. Insurance coverage varies, so ask about cost and whether it's routinely offered. For some people, the results bring understanding; for others, they don't change anything. There is no right reaction. The point is simply to know that this option exists and that you can ask for it if it would help you move forward.

Rhogam

If your blood type is Rh-negative, you may need an injection called Rhogam during or after a miscarriage to prevent complications in future pregnancies. Rhogam isn't about treating the miscarriage itself, it's about protecting against Rh sensitization, which can affect a future baby's red blood cells. Not everyone needs it, and timing matters: it's typically given within 72 hours of bleeding, pregnancy loss, or certain procedures. In some very early miscarriages, Rhogam may not be required, but many clinicians still recommend it out of caution. If no one has brought it up, you can ask directly, "Do I need Rhogam based on my blood type and how far along I was?"

If You Live in a Rural Area

Miscarriage care is especially complicated in rural communities, not because the people working there don't care, but because the system has stripped these hospitals of staff, specialists, and resources. Many rural hospitals struggle because of the following:

- Don't have an OB-GYN on site every day
- Rely on ER physicians who may have limited experience with miscarriage management
- Have no one credentialed to perform a D&C after hours
- Don't stock mifepristone due to regulation, fear, or pharmacy restrictions
- Have slow access to ultrasound, especially at night or on weekends
- Must transfer patients to larger hospitals for anything beyond basic stabilization

This means you may be told to "wait it out" not because it's the best option for you, but because it's the only option they *can* offer. That distinction matters.

In low-resource settings, the line between "appropriate expectant management" and "we can't provide anything else" gets blurry and patients aren't always told the truth about which one is happening.

Understanding this helps you ask clearer, safer questions such as the following:

- "Is expectant management the best option for me, or is it the only option available here today?"
- "Can this hospital manage complications if I need a procedure urgently?"
- "If I start bleeding heavier or show signs of infection, how fast can I be transferred?"
- "Is there a larger hospital within driving distance that offers full miscarriage management?"
- "If I need a D&C or emergency intervention, where would I go and how long would it take to get there?"

You're not overreacting. You're navigating care in a setting where the safety net has holes. Preparation and clarity can save time, and sometimes, save lives.

When (and Why) You Might Go to the ER

The majority of miscarriages don't *start* in the ER. They start at home. Spotting, cramps, a little blood. It can be hard to know when to watch and wait at home versus when to seek urgent care.

In general, the ER is the right place to go when you are worried about your safety. You might head to the ER if one of the following is true:

- Your bleeding is heavy, soaking through a pad in less than one to two hours.
- You feel dizzy, faint, weak, or your heart is racing.
- You have severe pain (especially sharp or one-sided) that isn't improving with medication.
- You pass very large clots (larger than a lemon).
- You have a fever, chills, or feel suddenly "off" or very sick.
- You have a history of ectopic pregnancy or your provider is worried about an ectopic but can't see you quickly.
- You can't reach any on-call clinician and you feel unsafe staying home.

When You're Being Sent Home and It Doesn't Feel Safe

If you're in the ER or urgent care and being sent home with "watch and wait" and it doesn't feel right, you are absolutely allowed to say so. You can slow things down. You can ask them to explain why. You can ask them to name what they are, and are not, willing to do. Try saying the following:

- "I want to understand all of my options—not just expectant management."
- "Is this plan based on my medical status, or on legal or institutional concerns?"
- "Can you document exactly why I'm being sent home, what my current symptoms are, and what options we discussed and declined?"
- "What specific signs should make me come back?"
- If you feel like you're being refused additional care, you can also say, "I'm requesting [medication management / a procedure/an obstetrician consult]. If that's not available or is being declined, please write in my chart that I requested it and that it was not provided, and explain why."

Asking these questions doesn't make you difficult. It creates a record. It signals that you understand what's happening.

And most important, it keeps you safer in a system that doesn't always default to your best interest.

A Note for Black Women and Birthing People

You shouldn't have to work twice as hard to be believed in the middle of a medical emergency. But we know the reality: Black patients experiencing miscarriage are more likely to be dismissed, delayed, or denied care, especially when they show up in pain or bleeding. Racism in medicine isn't just historical, it's happening right now, in ERs across the country.

Your pain is real. Your instincts are valid. You shouldn't have to "prove" how bad it is.

If you're being ignored or brushed off, you are *not* overreacting by pushing back or asking more questions. You're protecting your life.

You deserve care that takes your concerns seriously the first time. And you deserve providers who don't treat your miscarriage like a test of strength.

What Recovery Actually Looks Like (Physically and Emotionally)

Recovery is different for everyone, but here's what most people wish they'd been told up front. *Physically*, your body is coming down from pregnancy hormones while also healing from blood loss, cramping, and uterine changes. It's normal to have the following happen:

- Bleeding that tapers slowly over days to a couple of weeks
- Cramps that spike, then settle
- Spotting that comes and goes
- Fatigue that feels heavier than you expected
- Breast tenderness that lingers
- Mood swings driven by rapid hormone drops

None of these symptoms reflect how "far along" the pregnancy was. Your body responds to *hormonal change*, not gestational age.

Emotionally, you may feel grief, shock, relief, numbness, anger, or all of these in a single day. Some people feel connected to what they lost; others don't feel anything right away and wonder if that means something is "wrong." It doesn't. You're processing medical uncertainty and loss at the same time, which is an impossible double load.

You are allowed to rest. You are allowed to step back from work, childcare, or social plans. You don't need to power through this or pretend nothing happened. Your body just did something enormous. Your heart did, too.

A Final Word as You Move Through This

There is no "right" way to feel after a miscarriage. No timeline you're supposed to meet, no emotion you're supposed to have, no version of recovery that proves you're coping well enough. You've been navigating medical uncertainty, physical pain, and emotional overwhelm—often with little guidance and even less compassion from the system. That alone is a lot to carry. As you move forward, take what you need and leave what you don't: rest when you're tired, ask for help when you're overwhelmed, seek comfort wherever it finds you. Your loss is real, your experience is valid, and your body is not broken. You deserve care that meets you with clarity and dignity, not dismissal. And you deserve support that lasts longer than the bleeding does. Whatever comes next, whether you're grieving, healing, trying again, or simply trying to make sense of what happened, you don't have to go through it alone.

For Support People

They're experiencing pregnancy loss while potentially facing delayed care, dismissive treatment, or political interference in their medical care. They need someone to advocate fiercely for appropriate treatment and acknowledge their loss.

Acknowledging the loss. Even early miscarriage represents a real loss. Don't minimize it with "at least" statements or suggestions that they can "try again."

Advocating for care. Help them push for appropriate medical care rather than accepting "wait-and-see" approaches when they're in pain or bleeding heavily. Don't be polite if care is being delayed—be persistent and loud.

Managing logistics. Handle insurance issues, work communications, and follow-up appointments while they focus on physical and emotional recovery.

Fighting the system. In post-Dobbs healthcare, miscarriage care can be delayed or denied due to legal fears. Don't accept this. Demand immediate care, ask to speak to supervisors, and make it clear that delayed treatment is unacceptable. Document everything.

If you're joining for the visit. Advocate loudly for both pain management and bleeding management. Don't accept dismissive care or "wait and see" when they're bleeding heavily or in severe pain. Women have died from delayed miscarriage care due to abortion ban confusion. Don't let legal fears override medical necessity. Be the fierce advocate they need, demand action, and refuse to let them suffer while providers hesitate. Stand strong on their behalf, their life may depend on your willingness to make noise.

And if they're Black, the risks are even higher.

Racism in healthcare means Black women and birthing people are more likely to be ignored, misdiagnosed, or sent home too soon. They may not be believed about their pain, their bleeding, or their instincts, and that puts them at higher risk of harm. If you're supporting a Black loved one through miscarriage, your role as an advocate is even more critical.

Speak up when care is slow. Challenge bias when you see it.

Repeat their symptoms clearly. Ask direct questions. Make it clear you're watching. Ask for appropriate documentation if anything is denied. Ask to speak to the attending doctor. Ask for elevation to any supervisors. Remind providers that Black patients are more likely to suffer complications when their concerns are dismissed. Say it out loud if you need to: *"Black women are more likely to die from delayed miscarriage care. We're not taking that risk today."*

STRUCTURAL BARRIERS AND SAFETY NETS

Scenario 25

When You Don't Have Insurance

How to access reproductive care without coverage, what's legally protected, and how to find sliding scale support (especially helpful for undocumented patients, students, or gig workers)

There's a persistent myth in this country that if you don't have insurance, you're somehow disqualified from care. That myth is not only wrong, it's harmful. People lose insurance for all kinds of reasons: switching jobs, turning 26, losing a partner's plan, being undocumented, freelancing without benefits, living in a state that rejected Medicaid expansion, or simply not being able to afford the monthly premiums. And for some, especially undocumented patients or people in unsafe relationships, applying for coverage isn't just hard; it's risky.

None of that means you don't deserve care. None of that means you should be dismissed, shamed, or treated like a billing issue instead of a person.

You still have the right to understand your body. You still have the right to ask questions. You still have the right to protect your health—without apology.

This section breaks down two common realities:

- **I: You have insurance now but know you're about to lose it**, and you want to make the most of it while you still can.
- **II: You don't have insurance at all and aren't sure when, or if, you'll be able to get it.**

Wherever you fall, you deserve a plan you can actually use. Not guesswork. Not shame. Not "come back when you have insurance."

This is about giving you real tools to navigate a system that was never built with you in mind. It's about helping you access care safely, whether you're a student, a gig worker with unpredictable income, someone between jobs, or someone who can't safely apply for insurance at all.

Most of all, it's about reclaiming your power in a healthcare landscape that too often tries to take it from you.

Let's get you what you need.

I: If You're About to Lose Coverage

When insurance is ending, whether it's in two weeks or two months, what you do *now* can dramatically shape what the next chapter feels like. This is the moment to get the care that's free or affordable *today* and to set yourself up so you're not scrambling later.

Use Every Preventive Benefit While You Have Insurance

Preventive care is usually covered at 100%, even on high-deductible plans. This is the time to get anything that will be expensive or inaccessible without insurance:

- Pap smear
- Breast/chest exam or mammogram (if you're eligible)
- Sexually transmitted infection (STI) screening
- Blood pressure check and basic lab work (thyroid, A1C, cholesterol)
- Birth control counseling or refills

If you've been putting off these visits, get them now, they're the building blocks of reproductive care.

Consider Long-Acting Birth Control Before Your Plan Ends

If you want an intrauterine device or implant, now is the time. These are often fully covered, and they last 3–10 years depending on the type. Even if you're unsure about long-term plans, having a method in place can buy you stability during a period of financial or insurance transition when birth control may be out of reach.

Call Your Insurer for a Final Benefits Check

Ask directly:

- "Which preventive services are fully covered before my final date?"
- "Can I get extended medication refills now?"

Stock Up on Medications

Many plans allow 90-day refills; some allow up to a year of birth control if you request it. If your provider is willing, ask whether they can prescribe generics or longer refills to help you bridge the gap. Do they happen to have samples of your birth control pill? Even if cash-pay prices are low, stretching your current coverage helps.

Download Your Records Before You Lose Access

Before your final day of insurance download prior visit summaries, lab results, imaging reports, vaccines, and any past Pap or pathology results. You'll need these if you switch clinics or apply for financial assistance and when you're uninsured record retrieval can sometimes become harder than it should be.

Ask About Cash-Pay Pricing Now

If you plan to keep seeing the same clinic after your insurance ends, ask up front:

- "What are your self-pay rates?"
- "Do you have a sliding scale?"
- "Do you offer discounted lab packages for uninsured patients?"

Some clinics offer dramatically cheaper cash rates than people expect.

Losing coverage is stressful, but it doesn't have to leave you unprepared. A few strategic moves now can protect your health, and your wallet, for months to come.

II: If You're Uninsured

No insurance doesn't mean no care, it just means you may need a different plan. The system doesn't make this easy, but there *are* real, safe ways to get reproductive and general healthcare without coverage, and you deserve to know how to use them.

Low-Cost Clinics

Community health centers, Title X clinics, and public health departments exist *specifically* to care for people without insurance. They're legally required to offer confidential, sliding-scale services based on what you can afford. These clinics provide core reproductive care like birth control, Pap smears, STI testing/treatment, pregnancy tests, and basic OB-GYN visits. They also handle blood pressure checks and chronic disease screening. Some services, even Pap smears or contraception, may be completely free depending on funding.

Pharmacy and Online Access

Emergency contraception (like Plan B) is available over the counter, with no identification and no age requirement. In many states, pharmacists can prescribe birth control directly—pills, the patch, and the ring—saving you the cost of a clinic visit. Reputable telehealth platforms can also be a lifeline if transportation or clinic access is limited. For a flat fee, you can get care for urinary tract infections, yeast infections, birth control refills, or STI kits. Just make sure to read the fine print: some services add surprise fees for labs or follow-up messages.

Medication Assistance

Medications can be the biggest expense when you're uninsured, but there are ways to lower costs. Ask your provider or pharmacist about generic versions. They're often just as effective for a fraction of the price. Many major drug manufacturers offer patient assistance programs that can reduce medication costs dramatically, and many local pharmacies have their own discount cards or community programs you can use without signing up for insurance.

Being uninsured isn't a personal failure, it's a policy failure. And while the system might make you feel like you're supposed to disappear until you have coverage again, you still deserve care, dignity, and clear information. There *are* ways through this. Let's map them together.

Questions to Ask When You're Uninsured or Paying Out of Pocket

Start with basic pricing:

- "Is there a self-pay or uninsured rate?"
- "Do you offer a sliding scale based on income?"
- "Do you offer a discount for paying up front?"

Get clear costs before the visit begins:

- "Can I get a list of services and costs in advance?"
- "What is the cash price for this visit?"
- "Are there any additional fees I should be aware of?"

Before any labs or tests:

- "Which labs are necessary today—and what can wait?"
- "Can you tell me the cost of each lab before running them?"

If you need referrals or lower-cost options:

- "Are there any low-cost clinics nearby you'd recommend?"

Things to Watch Out For

Crisis Pregnancy Centers Pretending to be Clinics

These centers often target people without insurance by advertising "free ultrasounds" or "pregnancy support," but they *do not* provide medical care.

If a place doesn't offer contraception, STI testing, abortion referrals, or licensed clinicians, it's not a medical clinic. If they dodge questions or try to "counsel" you instead of giving clear answers, you can walk away.

Clinics That Can't Tell You What Anything Costs

When you're uninsured, transparency is nonnegotiable. A legitimate clinic will give you at least a price range for the visit and basic labs. If someone refuses to give any pricing over the phone, or keeps redirecting you, it's a red flag. You deserve to know what you're agreeing to before you walk in the door. Often clinics send swabs or tests that they've collected (Pap smears, STI testing, vaginal swabs) to a lab for processing.

The clinic may not know the pricing from the lab, but you can get the information for the lab to inquire yourself in advance of them sending it out. You can also ask for treatment based on assumption if you'd like to minimize lab test costs.

Surprise Tests You Didn't Ask For

Some clinics automatically add labs or procedures without explaining whether they're essential. When you're paying out of pocket, you can, and should, ask:

"Is this necessary today, or optional?"
"What happens if we skip this test?"
"What's the cost difference?"

Any provider who respects you will answer directly. If they can't explain why something is needed or the cost for it, that's your sign to slow things down.

Workbook: Mapping Your Care Without Insurance

Following is a practical guide to help you build a plan, protect your health, and stay in control—even when coverage is unstable or nonexistent.

What Preventive Care Do I Still Need?

List what you've had recently and what's overdue (Pap, STI testing, blood pressure check, thyroid, cholesterol, A1C, mammogram, vaccines):

Recent screenings/tests:

_____

_____

Still due/overdue:

_____

_____

_____

Medications to Refill or Plan For

Think through what you take regularly or occasionally (birth control, mental-health meds, asthma inhalers, thyroid meds, migraine meds, etc.).

Medications I need refilled now:

_____

_____

Medications I'll need soon:

_____

_____

Cash pay notes (prices, coupons, discount programs):

_____

_____

_____

Understanding My Healthcare Timeline

Coverage may return eventually. Planning around gaps helps you stay safe.

Do I expect to get coverage again?

☐ Yes *(when:* _____ *)*

☐ No/unsure

What care can safely wait until then?

_____

What care cannot wait?

_____

_____

What symptoms would make me go to urgent care or the ER?

_____

_____

_____

My Monthly Budget for Healthcare
Realistic monthly amount I can spend:

_____

My top priorities (birth control, mental-health meds, chronic disease meds, etc.):

_____

_____

Places to ask about payment plans or discounts:

_____

_____

Low-cost community labs or clinics to explore:

_____

_____

_____

For Support People

They're trying to access healthcare without insurance coverage, which creates additional stress and barriers on top of whatever health concerns brought them to seek care in the first place.

Reducing financial stress. Help research sliding-scale options, patient assistance programs, and community resources without making them feel ashamed about their insurance status.

Practical support. Offer specific help like transportation to distant clinics, childcare during appointments, or assistance with paperwork and applications.

Avoiding judgment. Don't lecture them about getting insurance or make assumptions about why they're uninsured. Focus on helping them get the care they need now.

If you're joining for the visit. Help them understand costs up front and advocate for transparent pricing and payment options.

Scenario 26

When You Live in a Rural Area

How to get reproductive care when the nearest clinic is hours away, telehealth is limited, and local options are few and far between

You're Not the Only One, Even If It Feels That Way

Living in a rural area often means you're used to stretching, improvising, and going without. Without a hospital nearby. Without specialists. Without reliable transportation options. And when it comes to reproductive healthcare, those gaps can leave you feeling like you're doing everything alone.

Maybe the OB-GYN you trusted retired. Maybe the nearest clinic doesn't take your insurance, or your concerns seriously. Maybe the only hospital left merged with a religious system that restricts contraception, miscarriage care, or gender-affirming care. Maybe the pharmacy across town frequently runs out of birth control or refuses to stock emergency contraception.

And here's the reality: the distance isn't the only barrier. Many rural hospitals have closed their labor and delivery units. Some have shut down altogether. Others can't keep providers because clinicians don't feel legally or professionally safe practicing full-scope reproductive care in hostile states.

That leaves *patients*, you, with fewer options, longer drives, and more risk.

This section helps you map what's available, plan for the gaps, and protect yourself medically and emotionally, even when the system offers you less.

You're not asking for too much. You're asking for basic healthcare in a place that may not have the resources to provide it.

When Clinics Are Hours Away or Don't Exist

Not every county has an OB-GYN. Some don't have a clinic offering Pap smears or sexually transmitted infection (STI) testing. Some don't have a pharmacy with reliable stock. It's not a personal failure; it's a policy failure. But you still deserve care.

Telehealth Options

Telehealth can fill gaps when states, systems, or broadband allow it.

What to ask locally:

- "Do you offer telehealth for follow-ups, medication refills, or birth control visits?"
- "Can we review labs or imaging by telehealth so I don't have to drive back?"
- "Can I start a visit by phone if video isn't reliable where I live?"

National platforms may offer the following service via telemed:

- Birth control prescriptions
- Urinary tract infection, yeast infection, and bacterial vaginosis treatment
- Menopausal symptom management
- Medication abortion by mail

Even if telehealth can't replace in-person care, it can reduce your trips, costs, and stress.

Pharmacy Access and Barriers

Rural pharmacies sometimes run out of stock or carry limited inventory. Some pharmacists have refused to fill birth control or emergency contraception based on personal or religious beliefs.

What helps:

- Ask the clinic to send prescriptions to the next closest pharmacy automatically.
- Call ahead to confirm a medication is in stock before driving.
- Ask, "Do you have an evening or weekend pickup window?"

In some states, pharmacists can prescribe birth control themselves, which can remove an entire visit from your to-do list.

Finding Providers Who Understand Rural Barriers

Certain clinics are specifically designed to serve rural patients:

- Federally qualified health centers
- Critical access hospitals
- Title X family planning clinics

They understand long drives, childcare constraints, weather, and the reality that you can't easily come back. When scheduling, try "Because I live *x* miles away, can we combine as much care as possible into one visit?"

Ask whether they can preorder labs, schedule imaging the same day, or do consults by phone before or after your appointment.

What Your Primary Care Provider Can Do (Even If There's No OB-GYN)

In many rural communities, your primary care provider (PCP) becomes your de facto reproductive health clinician. Most PCPs can safely provide the following:

- Pap smears and pelvic exams
- Birth control prescriptions (pills, patches, rings, shots)
- Intrauterine device (IUD) removal
- STI testing and treatment
- Pregnancy tests and early pregnancy counseling
- Perimenopause and menopause management
- Referrals for higher-level care

Some PCPs can also do the following:

- Place IUDs (long-acting reversible birth control placed in the uterus)
- Insert Nexplanon implants (a small hormonal rod placed in the arm for birth control)
- Manage uncomplicated miscarriage (early pregnancy loss without complications)
- Prescribe PrEP or PEP (medications to prevent HIV before or after possible exposure)
- Manage polycystic ovary syndrome, thyroid issues, or irregular cycles (common hormone-related conditions)

If you're unsure, ask directly, "Can you manage most of my reproductive care here, or do I need an OB-GYN for certain things?" This question alone can save you hours of driving.

Questions to Ask If You Live in a Rural Area

To combine care into fewer trips:

- "What services can you combine into one appointment so I don't have to drive back?"
- "Can I do labs locally and review results by telehealth or phone?"

To understand what's possible today:

- "If you don't offer this service, who does? And do I need a referral?"
- "Is there a larger hospital you partner with?"

For planning and safety:

- "Do you offer telehealth? What types of visits qualify?"
- "Are there mobile clinics serving my area soon?"
- "Is there a travel fund, gas reimbursement program, or voucher system available?"
- "What's your cancellation policy if I need to reschedule due to weather or transportation?"

To avoid unnecessary return trips:

- "Can we place standing orders for labs so I can do them at my local facility?"
- "Can you send my prescriptions to multiple pharmacies in case one doesn't stock them?"

Rural Pregnancy or Miscarriage Emergency Map

Living far from care means you need a plan before an emergency starts. Take a moment now to identify your closest emergency room (ER) (and how long the drive is during the day, at night, and in bad weather), whether that hospital has labor and delivery or an OB-GYN on call, and which larger hospital you'd go to if they don't. Know the closest clinic that offers pregnancy and miscarriage care—not just urgent care—and write down how to reach someone after hours. If 911 response is slow where you live, decide who your backup driver is. Learn your red flag symptoms so you don't second-guess yourself: heavy bleeding (soaking a pad in under one to two hours), dizziness or fainting, sharp or one-sided pelvic pain, fever with pelvic pain or foul discharge, or sudden severe symptoms later in pregnancy (vision changes, swelling, severe headache, right-sided abdominal pain). In rural areas, you don't wait to see if it gets worse—you go. Having this mapped out ahead of time isn't dramatic; it's what keeps you safe when care is distant, delayed, or limited.

Workbook: If You Live in a Rural Area

My nearest reproductive care options (distance / time):

_____

Telehealth services available in my state:

_____

My emergency plan (closest ER + backup):

_____

Transportation I can rely on:

_____

Questions I want to ask my clinician:

_____

For Support People

They're navigating reproductive healthcare in a place where resources are scarce, distances are long, and privacy isn't always guaranteed.

Offer practical support. Help drive to appointments, coordinate child-care, or assist with trip planning.

Help reduce the emotional load. Don't minimize the stress of distance or lack of access. Help them feel seen, not isolated.

Respect their privacy. In small towns, word travels fast. Be mindful about confidentiality and let them take the lead on sharing.

If you're joining for the visit. Be their backup. Help take notes, ask follow-up questions, and advocate for efficient care so they don't have to come back twice.

Scenario 27

Living in a State with an Abortion Ban

How to stay safe, protect your privacy, and navigate reproductive care when your state restricts or bans abortion

You Deserve Care, Even When the Law Says Otherwise

You shouldn't have to cross state lines to make a personal medical decision. But here you are, living in a place where abortion is banned, criminalized, or so restricted that access feels impossible. Maybe clinics have closed. Maybe hospitals refuse to treat anything that might be construed as abortion care. Maybe the rules keep shifting so quickly that you don't even know what's legal anymore.

And here's the hardest part: it's not just abortion that gets affected.

Miscarriage care, ectopic pregnancy care, prenatal care for complicated pregnancies, contraception access, even basic OB-GYN services, are now entangled with the same fear and confusion. The medications and procedures used for abortion (like mifepristone, misoprostol, and dilation and curettage) are the exact ones used for miscarriage and many pregnancy complications. When abortion is restricted, everything connected to it becomes slower, riskier, and less available.

You may feel isolated, scared to ask questions, or unsure where to turn.

You may feel like you have to justify your decisions to people who shouldn't get a say.

You may feel like your own body has become something the state is allowed to monitor or regulate.

But even in banned states, you still have options. You still have rights. You still deserve care.

What to Know Up Front

Here's the foundation you need before you make any decisions:

You do not have to justify your reasons. Whether this is a wanted pregnancy, an unwanted pregnancy, or a pregnancy you aren't sure about—you deserve care without explaining yourself to anyone.

Medication abortion is safe and effective. Mifepristone and misoprostol are used worldwide. They are also standard treatment for miscarriage. The science hasn't changed, the laws have.

Miscarriage and abortion care overlap:

The same medications
The same procedures
The same clinicians

That overlap is why bans have made miscarriage care so unsafe.

Legal Risk: What to Know, What to Ask

You don't need to memorize the laws in your state—most are intentionally confusing and change faster than any patient could keep track of. What you *can* do is anchor yourself in practices that protect your privacy and your safety while you navigate a system that doesn't always feel trustworthy. Start by relying on reputable legal hotlines rather than social media; they monitor the law in real time so you don't have to live in a constant state of fear or guessing.

Protecting your digital footprint also matters. Use private browsing if you can, delete searches afterward, avoid holding onto pill packaging, and consider using encrypted apps when talking about sensitive care. These steps aren't about hiding wrongdoing, they're about keeping yourself safe in a landscape where misunderstanding can quickly lead to scrutiny.

If you used abortion medications and are now seeking follow-up care, you're allowed to use medically accurate language that protects your privacy. Saying "I think I'm having a miscarriage" is truthful, clinically appropriate, and gives providers the information they need.

There is *no* blood test, urine test, or ultrasound that can distinguish a spontaneous miscarriage from a medication abortion. The only physical difference is that misoprostol placed vaginally can sometimes leave detectable residue for four to five days. This is why many people in restricted states choose to use it buccally (in the cheek), where no residue remains and nothing is detectable on exam. Either way, you are not required to provide details that put you at risk or make you feel unsafe.

And above all: trust your instincts. If a provider's tone shifts, if questions feel more investigative than clinical, or if something in the interaction makes you uneasy, you're allowed to slow down, offer only the medical information necessary for treatment, or pause until you can reach legal support. You don't owe anyone a story that compromises your safety.

Caution: Where Not to Go

In states with abortion bans, the difference between safe care and harmful care can be subtle but deeply important. Some places exist to support you; others exist to delay, shame, or block you from getting the care you need. Crisis pregnancy centers, often disguised as real clinics, are designed to stall you, discourage abortion in any form, and rarely offer actual medical services. Other settings may quietly refuse miscarriage treatment until you're sicker, insisting they "can't intervene yet" even when you're bleeding heavily or in pain. And some spaces wrap their care in religious pressure, moralizing language, or vague legal warnings meant to scare you into silence.

If you feel judged, unsafe, or interrogated, you're allowed to walk out.

If someone tries to guilt you or withhold information, you can leave.

What This Means for *All* of Reproductive Healthcare (It's All Connected)

Abortion bans don't exist in isolation. They reshape the entire reproductive health landscape around them. Even if you never seek an abortion, here's how bans may affect *your* care:

- **Contraception access becomes harder.** Some pharmacies refuse to stock emergency contraception. Some clinicians avoid prescribing intrauterine devices for fear they'll be accused of providing abortion care.
- **Miscarriage care becomes delayed.** Doctors hesitate to offer mifepristone, even when it's the safest option. Hospitals require legal review before treating patients. People are sent home bleeding.
- **High-risk prenatal care becomes inconsistent or unavailable.** Maternal fetal medicine specialists leave hostile states. Hospitals close obstetrics units. Pregnant patients have fewer providers and fewer specialists.
- **Ectopic pregnancy treatment gets delayed.** Fear of "terminating a pregnancy" makes some clinicians stall, even though untreated ectopic pregnancies are life-threatening emergencies.
- **People with chronic conditions struggle to get medications.** Drugs like methotrexate (used for rheumatoid arthritis) become harder to fill because they can also end a pregnancy.
- **Patients get sicker. Some die.** This isn't theoretical. It's happening now.

Understanding that all reproductive care is connected helps you see your risk more clearly and helps you plan ahead, advocate earlier, and get support faster.

You aren't imagining it. You aren't overreacting. The system is failing, but you don't have to face it alone.

See Other Scenarios That Might Help

If you're navigating care in a state with abortion bans, you may find these sections especially relevant:

Scenario 24: Miscarriage Management. For a deeper look at how miscarriage and abortion care overlap, why care is being delayed or denied in banned states, and the exact language and scripts you can use to advocate for yourself in an emergency room (ER)

Scenario 26: When You Live in a Rural Area. For guidance on traveling long distances for care, planning around limited clinic access, using telehealth strategically, and building an emergency backup plan when local options are scarce

---

For Support People

They may be facing a pregnancy they can't continue—or a miscarriage they can't complete safely—because the system failed them. It's not just logistics. It's grief, fear, and shame they never should've had to carry.

Help them feel seen. You don't have to fix it—just show up. Let them cry, rage, vent, or sit in silence. Be the person who doesn't look away.

Protect their privacy. Don't share what's happening unless they've asked you to. Be mindful of who's in the room, what's in writing, and how things are stored or shared.

Offer real-world support. Help with research, travel plans, recovery care, or even just packing a bag. Concrete help goes a long way.

Check in later. Even if they say they're okay, follow up. Being denied care can leave lasting trauma—especially if they were dismissed, mistreated, or made to feel unsafe.

If you're going with them. Be their calm, their advocate, their witness. Whether it's a long drive or a quiet night at home after taking pills, your presence matters. And if they land in the ER for miscarriage care or pain, your voice might be the one that gets them help. Speak up. Push back. Refuse to be ignored.

Scenario 28

Navigating Reproductive Coercion, Abuse, or Control

How to protect your body, your choices, and your safety when someone else is trying to control your reproductive decisions

Note to the Reader

I wasn't sure whether to include this section in the book. It's heavy. It's hard. And it's not something we talk about enough. But if this book is about helping people advocate for themselves, *really* advocate, then I would be wrong to leave this out. I hope it helps. Even just one person.

This section is for the moments that are harder to name. When the issue isn't just access or insurance or provider fit, but control. When someone else is making decisions about your body, your privacy, or your pregnancy. Sometimes it's obvious, sometimes we don't realize until it's too late.

If this section resonates, you are not alone. And you deserve safety, care, and autonomy—no matter what anyone else has told you.

There are other organizations and support systems that are far better equipped to help with the full picture: emergency housing, financial safety planning, legal aid, protective services, and trauma recovery. But the purpose of this scenario, and this book, is to focus on the part of the picture that's often missed: the reproductive healthcare.

Just like the other scenarios in this workbook, this one is here to help you *advocate for yourself*, especially when you're not safe or free to do so openly. You don't need to tell your whole story. But you still deserve the information, language, and support to protect your body and your choices.

What Reproductive Coercion Can Look Like

You don't need to have someone do every one of these. Even just a few can be harmful:

- Pressuring you to become pregnant or continue a pregnancy
- Forcing or threatening you to end a pregnancy
- Hiding, destroying, or interfering with birth control
- Refusing to use protection or sabotaging condoms
- Denying or restricting access to OB-GYN visits
- Requiring access to your patient portal or test results
- Forcing you to take medications or undergo procedures
- Tracking your phone, cycle, or location
- Threatening to share intimate images or health info
- Using pregnancy as a method of control or dependency
- Refusing to let you speak privately with a provider

You Can Plan for Safety Without Disclosing Abuse

If you're not ready, or not able, to disclose what's happening, you can still take steps to protect yourself:

- Use private or incognito browsers to search for care.
- Set up a second email that only you can access for health info / request that appointment reminders not be sent to certain numbers or emails.
- Use cash for appointments when possible to avoid paper trails.
- Call clinics in advance and ask, "Can I have a private moment alone with the provider?" or "Can I leave a note in my chart?"
- Avoid logging into patient portals on shared devices.
- Ask to speak with the provider alone, even if someone insists on staying with you. You can say, "I have a sensitive question I'd prefer to ask privately."

- Ask how to document abuse for potential legal proceedings.
- Use code words with trusted friends or family if needed. Example: "If I say I'm ordering pizza, I need help."

What You Can Say in the Exam Room

Even a single sentence can open the door to support. You don't have to tell the full story.

- "I don't feel safe in my relationship, and I need help protecting my reproductive choices."
- "Someone's pressuring me about pregnancy decisions, and I don't want them to know I'm here."
- "Can I speak with you alone, without anything showing in the portal?"
- "I need discreet care. Can you help me with that?"

Questions to Ask Your Provider (or Yourself)

- "Can we discuss birth control options that no one else can detect or control?"
- "Can I opt out of online access or change how communications are sent?"
- "Is it safe for me to list this visit on my insurance, or should we talk about other options?"
- "Can this be noted in the chart without others seeing it?"
- "If I'm being pressured or controlled, what support is there?"

Safer Birth Control Options When Privacy Matters

- **Intrauterine devices and implants.** These can't be seen, and may not be felt externally.
- **Depo-Provera shot.** One injection every three months provides protection, without pills to hide.
- **Emergency contraception.** Some brands are available over the counter and without identification.
- **Cycle tracking apps.** Avoid apps that share data; look for privacy-first or paper options.
- **No method** is 100% undetectable, but providers can help you choose based on your situation.

If You're in Immediate Danger or Think You're Being Trafficked

You don't have to figure this out alone. Help exists. You deserve to access it safely, on your own terms. At the time this book was written, these were the national resources available:

- **National Domestic Violence Hotline**

  Call **800–799–SAFE (7233)** or go to thehotline.org.
  It's confidential and they can help you safety plan, understand your options, and get connected to local resources.

- **National Human Trafficking Hotline**

  Call **888–373–7888** or go to humantraffickinghotline.org.
  You don't need proof to reach out. You don't have to know whether what's happening "counts." They will listen and help you navigate next steps.

In the exam room, you can simply say, "I need help leaving safely. Can you connect me to someone?"

You don't have to tell your whole story. You don't have to justify your fear. You don't have to be ready to leave for your safety to matter.

Even if you aren't ready, or able, to disclose everything, you are still allowed to get care that prioritizes your well-being.

A Final Word: You Deserve Safety, Autonomy, and Care

Reproductive coercion is one of the most hidden forms of abuse because it sits at the intersection of health, relationships, and control. It's not always loud or obvious. Sometimes it looks like pressure disguised as love, "concern" that's really surveillance, or support that quietly erases your choices. Other times it's violent, threatening, or unmistakably controlling. None of it is your fault.

If anything in this section feels familiar, take a breath.

You are not overreacting. You are not imagining it. You are not "being dramatic" or "making it up."

You are naming something that many people go through in silence.

And I want to be clear: I understand this isn't simple. Leaving isn't always safe. Disclosing isn't always possible. Relationships can be complicated, layered, and tied to housing, finances, children, culture, community, and survival. Nothing about this is black-and-white. Nothing about this is easy. Complexity doesn't make your situation less real.

You still deserve care that centers *you*, your safety, your decisions, your future. Even if you can't openly disclose what's happening. Even if someone is monitoring your phone, controlling your movements, or sitting in the room with you. Even if you're not ready to leave.

This scenario isn't here to tell you what to do. It's here to give you options when someone else has tried to take yours away. It's here so you have language, strategies, and a way forward that protects your body and your autonomy.

And if this chapter is the first time you've seen your situation reflected anywhere, I am so glad you found it.

You deserve privacy. You deserve compassion. You deserve control over your reproductive health. You deserve to be safe, on your own terms, in your own time. And you are not alone.

For Support People

If someone shares that they're being pressured, tracked, or coerced—believe them and stay with them.

- **Believe what they say,** even if it's confusing or fragmented.
- **Help without pushing**—let them set the pace for safety or change.
- **Offer logistical help,** like researching clinics, creating new logins, or covering private transportation.
- **Don't lecture or interrogate**—even if you're scared for them.
- **If they're ready for help.** Offer to connect them with a domestic violence hotline, legal advocate, or social worker who specializes in reproductive abuse or trafficking.

Your presence and patience may be the lifeline they need to take their next step safely.

You Made It Through
the Hard Part

Now You're Walking In with More Than Just Questions.
You've just moved through some of the hardest conversations we *never* get handed scripts for. Miscarriage. Coercion. Menopause. Trying to get pregnant. Trying not to. Standing in a broken system with nothing but a paper gown and a pounding heart. And learning how to speak anyway.

You learned how to ask the real questions. How to spot red flags. How to prepare before the visit and recover after the hard ones. How to advocate not just with knowledge, but with care.

But most important? You learned that you're allowed to take up space.

That you're not too loud. Not too complicated. Not too late.

That even when the system tries to make you small, you still belong.

These aren't just scenarios. They're blueprints. For advocating in real time. For protecting your peace. For knowing that your pain, your joy, your body, and your future all matter—and deserve care that reflects that.

No, this book didn't teach you everything.

You might still have questions. Unfortunately, this book couldn't cover it all.

But hopefully it helped you learn how to ask. How to push when you're being brushed off. How to stay in your body when someone tries to talk over it. How to get the information you need, even when the system makes it hard. How not to shrink when they try to make you smaller. How to stand your ground. How to get what you need.

Come back when you need it. Mark the pages that serve you. Share them with someone you love.

And remember:

You don't have to have all the answers.

You just have to know you deserve better.

You do.

We do.

We deserve more.

Printed and bound by CPI Group (UK) Ltd, Croydon, CR0 4YY

28/04/2026

14869806-0002